T0348598

The Cavus Foot

Editor

ALEXEJ BARG

FOOT AND ANKLE CLINICS

www.foot.theclinics.com

Consulting Editor
MARK S. MYERSON

June 2019 • Volume 24 • Number 2

ELSEVIER

1600 John F. Kennedy Boulevard ● Suite 1800 ● Philadelphia, Pennsylvania, 19103-2899

http://www.theclinics.com

FOOT AND ANKLE CLINICS Volume 24, Number 2
June 2019 ISSN 1083-7515, ISBN-978-0-323-68208-4

Editor: Lauren Boyle
Developmental Editor: Meredith Madeira

Foot and Ankle Clinics (ISSN 1083-7515) is published quarterly by Elsevier, Inc., 360 Park Avenue South, New York, NY 10010-1710. Months of issue are March, June, September, and December. Periodicals postage paid at New York, NY, and additional mailing offices. Subscription price per year is $337.00 (US individuals), $552.00 (US institutions), $100.00 (US students), $371.00 (Canadian individuals), $663.00 (Canadian institutions), $215.00 (Canadian students), $465.00 (international individuals), $663.00 (international institutions), and $215.00 (international students). To receive student/resident rate, orders must be accompanied by name of affiliated institution, date of term, and the *signature* of program/residency coordinator on institution letterhead. Orders will be billed at individual rate until proof of status is received. Foreign air speed delivery is included in all *Clinics* subscription prices. All prices are subject to change without notice. **POSTMASTER:** Send address changes to *Foot and Ankle Clinics*, Elsevier Health Sciences Division, Subscription Customer Service, 3251 Riverport Lane, Maryland Heights, MO 63043. **Customer Service: 1-800-654-2452 (US and Canada). From outside of the United States and Canada, call 314-447-8871. Fax: 314-447-8029. E-mail: JournalsCustomerService-usa@elsevier.com (for print support); JournalsOnlineSupport-usa@elsevier.com (for online support).**

Reprints. For copies of 100 or more, of articles in this publication, please contact the Commercial Reprints Department, Elsevier Inc., 360 Park Avenue South, New York, NY 10010-1710. Tel.: 212-633-3874; Fax: 212-633-3820; E-mail: reprints@elsevier.com.

Editorial Advisory Board

Contributors

CONSULTING EDITOR

MARK S. MYERSON, MD
Medical Director, The Foot and Ankle Association, Inc, Baltimore, Maryland, USA

EDITOR

ALEXEJ BARG, MD
Assistant Professor, Department of Orthopaedics, University of Utah, Salt Lake City, Utah, USA

AUTHORS

CRAIG C. AKOH, MD
Sports Medicine Fellow, Department of Orthopedics and Rehabilitation, University of Wisconsin School of Medicine and Public Health Madison, Madison, Wisconsin, USA

FAISAL ALSAYEL, MD
Orthopaedic Fellow, Swiss Ortho Center, Schmerzklinik Basel, Swiss Medical Network, Basel, Switzerland

ALEXEJ BARG, MD
Assistant Professor, Department of Orthopaedics, University of Utah, Salt Lake City, Utah, USA

STEVEN L. HADDAD, MD
Senior Attending Orthopaedic Surgeon, Illinois Bone and Joint Institute, LLC, Glenview, Illinois, USA

BEAT HINTERMANN, MD
Associate Professor and Chairman, Clinic of Orthopaedic Surgery, Kantonsspital Baselland, Liestal, Switzerland

NICOLA KRÄHENBÜHL, MD
Department of Orthopaedics, Research Fellow, University of Utah, Salt Lake City, Utah, USA

FABIAN KRAUSE, MD
Department of Orthopaedic Surgery, Inselspital, University of Berne, Berne, Switzerland

SHUYUAN LI, MD, PhD
Program Coordinator, Steps2Walk, Baltimore, Maryland, USA

LUIGI MANZI, MD
C.A.S.C.O. Foot and Ankle Unit, IRCCS Galeazzi, Milan, Italy

C. LUCAS MYERSON, BA
Tulane University School of Medicine, New Orleans, Louisiana, USA

MARK S. MYERSON, MD
Medical Director, The Foot and Ankle Association, Inc, Baltimore, Maryland, USA

JULIE A. NEUMANN, MD
Fellow, Department of Orthopaedics, University of Utah, University Orthopaedic Center, Salt Lake City, Utah, USA

FLORIAN NICKISCH, MD
Associate Professor, Department of Orthopaedics, University of Utah, University Orthopaedic Center, Salt Lake City, Utah, USA

PHINIT PHISITKUL, MD
Orthopaedic Surgeon, Tri-State Specialists, LLP, Sioux City, Iowa, USA

AKARADECH PITAKVEERAKUL, MD
Department of Orthopaedic Surgery, Sirindhorn Hospital, Bangkok Metropolitan Administration, Bangkok, Thailand

STEFAN RAMMELT, MD, PhD
Professor, University Center for Orthopaedics and Traumatology, University Hospital Carl-Gustav Carus at TU Dresden, Dresden, Germany

ROXA RUIZ, MD
Senior Attending Foot and Ankle Surgeon, Clinic of Orthopaedic Surgery, Kantonsspital Baselland, Liestal, Switzerland

CHARLES L. SALTZMAN, MD
Louis S. Peery Endowed Presidential Professor, Chairman, Department of Orthopaedics, University of Utah, Salt Lake City, Utah, USA

BRIAN STEGINSKY, DO
Attending Orthopedic Surgeon, OhioHealth Orthopedic Surgeons, Columbus, Ohio, USA

FEDERICO GIUSEPPE USUELLI, MD
C.A.S.C.O. Foot and Ankle Unit, IRCCS Galeazzi, Milan, Italy

VICTOR VALDERRABANO, MD, PhD
Chairman, Swiss Ortho Center, Professor, University of Basel, Schmerzklinik Basel, Swiss Medical Network, Basel, Switzerland

MAXWELL W. WEINBERG, BS
Department of Orthopaedics, Research Coordinator, University of Utah, Salt Lake City, Utah, USA

KAI ZIEBARTH, MD
Department of Pediatric Surgery, Inselspital, University of Berne, Berne, Switzerland

Contents

A high longitudinal plantar arch, varus position of the heel, forefoot equinus, and pronation of the first ray are characteristic of a cavovarus deformity. Forefoot-driven and hindfoot-driven deformities are distinguished based on pathomechanics. In first ray strong plantarflexion, the forefoot touches the ground first. This leads to compensatory varus heel, lock of the midfoot, reduction of the flexible phase, and decrease in shock absorption. In hindfoot-driven cavovarus deformity, the subtalar joint may compensate for varus deformities above the ankle joint. Overload of the lateral soft tissue structures and degenerative changes may occur in longstanding cavovarus deformity.

The purpose of the clinical examination is to detect subtle cavus or cavovarus deformity, assess the severity and type of deformity, differentiate between idiopathic versus secondary etiologies of cavus foot deformity, and evaluate for other associated abnormalities. The clinical examination should begin with a gait analysis. The neurologic examination reveals peripheral neuropathy or central nervous system etiology for the foot deformity. On plain radiographs, forefoot-driven deformity can be assessed using the Meary angle, and hindfoot-driven deformity can be measured by the calcaneal pitch. Computed tomography and MRI scans can assess for tarsal coalitions and soft tissue pathologies, respectively.

A cavovarus deformity results from muscle imbalances in the foot. There are several etiologies of a cavovarus foot including congenital, neurologic, post-traumatic, and idiopathic. Charcot-Marie-Tooth disease is a common genetic cause of cavovarus foot. History, physical examination, and imaging help determine appropriate treatment. The deformity can be flexible or rigid and can present in children or adults, thus treatment should be individualized to the patient. Non-operative management includes shoe wear modification, physical therapy, and bracing. Operative management consists of soft tissue releases, tendon transfers, osteotomies, arthrodesis, and repair/reconstruction of lateral ankle ligaments and peroneal tendons.

The treatment goal for pediatric cavovarus deformities is to neutralize plantar pressure distribution, reduce hindfoot varus deformity, and avoid or postpone ankle, midfoot, and hindfoot arthritis. If nonoperative treatment is not sufficient, surgical realignment must be discussed. Promising improvements in decision making and operative techniques have been published. To avoid disappointment owing to recurrence or failures of operative procedures, selection of the appropriate and preferably single operative procedure remains the most crucial factor for success. This article focuses on current treatment options depending on the localization of the anatomic pathology. Outcomes of nonoperative and operative treatments are presented.

The cavo varus foot is a complex pathology due to skeletal deformity and neuro-muscular unbalance. The key concept for a successful treatment is to consider the whole foot and ankle complex from a bone and soft tissue perspective. Undercorrection is the main issue in cavo varus foot management, which may be attributed to intrinsic correction defects of the described calcaneal osteotomies or to a lack of understanding about the pathology and the subsequent algorithm of treatment. The authors disclose their daily algorithm of treatment, considering the foot and ankle complex and the role of calcaneal osteotomies in ankle inframalleolar deformities.

The most common cause for end-stage ankle osteoarthritis is posttraumatic, sometimes resulting from concomitant supramalleolar deformity. Aims of the supramalleolar osteotomy include restoring the lower-leg axis to improve intraarticular load distribution and retarding degeneration of the tibiotalar joint. Preoperative planning is based on conventional weight-bearing radiographs. Often advanced imaging, including computed tomography and/or MRI, is needed for a better understanding of the underlying problem. Postoperative complications are not uncommon, including progression of tibiotalar osteoarthritis in up to 25% within 5 years of all patients who have supramalleolar osteotomies.

Patients with varus ankle deformity and concomitant osteoarthritis experience severe disabling pain that affects their daily activity of living. Most cases rarely respond to nonoperative treatment. One surgical option is corrective ankle arthrodesis. Unfortunately, this corrective surgery is challenging and might not be possible as a purely isolated procedure. Corrective ankle arthrodesis for varus ankle is performed with different surgical approaches and techniques, using different methods of fixations. The goal of surgery is to create a pain-free, stable, and plantigrade ankle, hindfoot, and foot. Both the foot and ankle must be correctly aligned in the optimal position for proper locomotion.

Coronal plane deformity following total ankle arthroplasty has been associated with poor clinical outcomes and early prosthesis failure. Neutral mechanical alignment and prosthetic joint stability must be achieved through meticulous surgical planning and precise technical execution. Cavovarus foot deformity and varus malalignment of the lower extremity is reviewed, with particular emphasis as it relates to total ankle arthroplasty. Correction of varus malalignment may be performed at the time of total ankle arthroplasty or as a 2-stage procedure. Surgeon experience, revision total ankle arthroplasty, and subtalar arthrodesis should be considerations when contemplating 2-stage varus correction.

In the past few decades, total ankle replacement (TAR) has become an increasingly recommended and accepted treatment in patients with end-stage ankle osteoarthritis. However, controversy still exists about the appropriate indications for TAR, specifically in ankles with coronal plane deformities. Although not explicitly proved, the long-term success of TAR seems to largely depend on the extent to which the surgeon is able to balance the ankle joint complex.

Posttraumatic hindfoot varus may result from nonoperative treatment or inadequate reduction and fixation of talar and calcaneal fractures. Adequate visualization of the talar neck via bilateral approaches is essential in avoiding malreduction. In cases of medial comminution of the talar neck, lag screws must be avoided and the use of single or double plates should be considered. A Schanz screw introduced into the calcaneal tuberosity is instrumental in realigning shortening, varus, or valgus deformity of the heel. Special attention should be paid to addressing impaction of the medial facet of both the talus and calcaneus to avoid hindfoot varus.

Mild to moderate cavus deformity creates a dilemma in terms of surgical decision-making. The decision to pursue osteotomy or arthrodesis is not always clear. This article provides a framework for guiding management of these deformities, followed by a detailed surgical approach to correcting moderate cavus deformities, which emphasizes the use of a midfoot osteotomy-arthrodesis.

Recurrent deformity after surgical treatment of the cavus foot occurs because a procedure is not performed at the apex of the deformity. In many instances there are multiple apices and, in addition to hindfoot osteotomy or arthrodesis, the midfoot must be corrected. There is not much of a role for the Coleman block test to determine flexibility of the foot, and this has led to many failures where the foot was believed flexible and an osteotomy was insufficient treatment. Skeletal correction, even if perfect, does not last unless the foot is balanced with appropriate tendon transfers.

FOOT AND ANKLE CLINICS

RELATED INTEREST

Clinics in Podiatric Medicine and Surgery, January 2018 (Vol. 35, No. 1)
New Technologies in Foot and Ankle Surgery
Stephen A. Brigido, *Editor*
https://www.podiatric.theclinics.com/

THE CLINICS ARE NOW AVAILABLE ONLINE!
Access your subscription at:
www.theclinics.com

Preface
The Cavus Foot

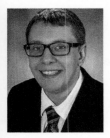

Alexej Barg, MD
Editor

Surgical management of the cavovarus deformity remains one of the biggest challenges in foot and ankle surgery. The already complex anatomy and biomechanics of the foot and ankle are further obfuscated when a cavovarus deformity develops and worsens over time. Several treatment algorithms, which are more or less complicated tables and diagrams, have been published over the last few decades. However, such "cookbook" solutions should be interpreted carefully; "standard" procedures often need to be modified due to the complexity and uniqueness of each case. The overall goal of this issue is not to provide another "structured treatment algorithm," but rather to highlight the importance of an exact understanding and diagnosis of the underlying cavovarus deformity and to share personal experiences on its surgical treatment.

It has become a great tradition for every issue of *Foot and Ankle Clinics of North America* to be prepared by experts in their field from all over the world. I was lucky enough to be able to carry on this international spirit and collaborate with colleagues who are renowned experts in foot and ankle surgery and who have agreed to share their knowledge with all of us. I would like to commend all of the authors of this issue on their excellent work and the enormous amount of time and effort devoted to preparing each article. I would like to thank Meredith Madeira from Elsevier for her adept technical and editorial support. And, of course, my special thanks goes to Mark S. Myerson, MD, for his kind invitation to be the guest editor of this issue. He gave me the freedom to shape the content of this issue, and our

Foot Ankle Clin N Am 24 (2019) xiii–xiv
https://doi.org/10.1016/j.fcl.2019.02.013
1083-7515/19/© 2019 Published by Elsevier Inc.

discussions together provided invaluable guidance. I hope you enjoy reading this month's issue!

Alexej Barg, MD
Department of Orthopaedics
University of Utah
590 Wakara Way
Salt Lake City, UT 84108, USA

E-mail address:
alexej.barg@hsc.utah.edu

Anatomy and Biomechanics of Cavovarus Deformity

Nicola Krähenbühl, MD*, Maxwell W. Weinberg, BS

KEYWORDS

- Cavovarus deformity • Heel pain • Coleman block test • Biomechanics

KEY POINTS

- Cavovarus deformity can be the result of a plantar flexed first ray (forefoot-driven), a deformity of the hindfoot (hindfoot-driven), or a combination of both.
- In midstance, plantarflexion of the first ray leads to a compensatory varus heel, a lock in the midfoot, and reduced shock absorption.
- During heel-off (terminal stance), the plantarflexed first ray causes a supination of the forefoot that increases the varus deformity of the hindfoot.
- In hindfoot-driven cavovarus deformity, the subtalar joint may compensate for varus deformities above the ankle joint.
- Overload of the lateral soft tissue structures (eg, lateral ligament complex, peroneal tendons) and degenerative changes (eg, medial ankle osteoarthritis, midfoot arthritis) may occur over time.

INTRODUCTION

Cavovarus deformity is characterized by a high longitudinal plantar arch, varus position of the heel, forefoot equinus, and pronation of the first ray in stance (**Fig. 1**).[1–3] Based on the pathomechanics, cavovarus deformity can be the result of a plantar flexed first ray (forefoot-driven), a deformity of the hindfoot (hindfoot-driven), or a combination of both.[1,4,5] The etiologic factors of cavovarus deformity are not uniform. If bilateral, neurologic diseases such as hereditary motor and sensory neuropathies and congenital deformities (eg, rotational deformities, residual clubfoot) are common reasons for a cavovarus deformity (**Fig. 2**). A unilateral presentation is typical for posttraumatic conditions (eg, pilon fracture, talus neck fracture).[1,5–7] In some cases, the underlying primary cause cannot be determined (idiopathic).[6] In the case of an underlining neurologic disease, the deformity is most frequently caused by a muscle imbalance.[1] In posttraumatic conditions, however, cavovarus deformity is often the result of posttraumatic bony deformities and/or ligamentous instability.[4,5] Although cavovarus

Department of Orthopaedics, University of Utah, 590 Wakara Way, Salt Lake City, UT 84108, USA
* Corresponding author.
E-mail address: nicola.krahenbuhl@hsc.utah.edu

Foot Ankle Clin N Am 24 (2019) 173–181
https://doi.org/10.1016/j.fcl.2019.02.001
1083-7515/19/© 2019 Elsevier Inc. All rights reserved.

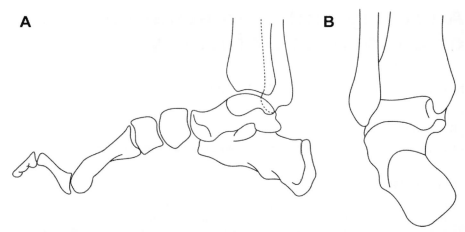

Fig. 1. Characteristics of the cavovarus deformity. (*A*) Medial view. The distance between the calcaneus and the metatarsal heads is reduced and the medial arch is elevated. Hyperextension of the metatarsal-phalangeal joint and flexion of the interphalangeal joint are present. The fibula is slightly posteriorly rotated. (*B*) Hindfoot alignment. The heel is in varus position.

deformity can be initially compensated, it may become more rigid over time. In the case of premature bone growth, a cavovarus deformity affects the further development of the bones, leading to alteration of their shape and morphology.[8] In adults, the influence of cavovarus deformity on bony morphology is minor.[9] Overload of the lateral soft tissue structures (eg, lateral ligament complex, peroneal tendons) and degenerative changes (eg, medial ankle osteoarthritis, midfoot arthritis) may occur over time.[4] This article highlights the anatomic and biomechanical characteristics of cavovarus deformity.

FOREFOOT-DRIVEN CAVOVARUS DEFORMITY

Forefoot-driven cavovarus deformity is frequently caused by an underlying neurologic disease (**Table 1**).[3,5] In this case, the deformity is the result of an imbalance between

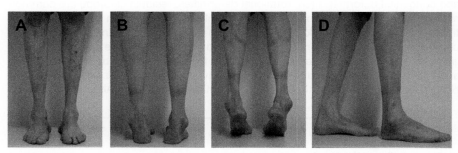

Fig. 2. Neurologic cavovarus deformity. (*A*) The heel pad is prominent when viewed from the front (peek-a-boo sign). (*B*) Evaluation from the back showing a distinct hindfoot varus alignment. (*C*) During heel-off, supination of the forefoot occurs and a more distinct hindfoot varus alignment is evident. (*D*) Elevation of the medial arch and a shortened medial column are visible from the lateral view. In addition, the lateral part of the foot is overloaded.

Table 1		
Etiologic factors of cavovarus deformity		
Neurologic	Trauma	Others
• HMSN (eg, CMT disease)	• Compartment syndrome	• Tarsal coalition
• Spinal tumors	• Short-foot syndrome	• Rotational deformities
• Spinal dysraphism	• Scar tissue	• Residual clubfoot
• Cerebral palsy	• Burns	• Idiopathic
• Poliomyelitis	• Vascular lesions	• Rheumatoid arthritis
• Myelomeningocele	• Hindfoot instability	• Ankle osteoarthritis
• Polyneuritic syndromes	• Tibial fracture	• Plantar fibromatosis
• Stroke	• Talar neck fracture	• Varus subtalar joint axis
• Parkinson	• Calcaneal fracture	• Diabetic foot syndrome

Abbreviations: CMT, charcot-marie-tooth; HMSN, hereditary motor and sensory neuropathy.

agonistic and antagonistic muscles.[5] In particular, the peroneus longus, peroneus brevis, tibialis anterior, and tibialis posterior muscles were identified to have a major influence on the development of a cavovarus deformity.[1,10] Because the peroneus longus muscle has various insertions at the metatarsals and medial cuneiform, overdrive of the peroneus longus causes plantarflexion of the first ray.[1,11] Muscular imbalance, including weakness of the tibialis anterior and peroneus brevis muscles, combined with a strong tibialis posterior muscle can lead to the characteristic changes of a cavovarus deformity over time.[1,5] Typically, the forefoot is in pronation (midstance), the midfoot is in supination, the medial longitudinal arch is elevated, and the medial column is shortened.[1] The foot is adducted and the distance between the navicular bone and the floor is increased, whereas the distance between the calcaneal tuberosity and the metatarsal heads is decreased.[1] To compensate for the forefoot deformity (plantar flexed first ray), the hindfoot adopts a varus position.[1] Therefore, forefoot-driven cavovarus deformities do not only involve the forefoot but also the midfoot and hindfoot (**Fig. 3**).

Due to hyperactivity of the long flexors, a cock-up deformity of the metatarsalphalangeal (MTP) joints and clawing of the proximal and distal interphalangeal joints develop.[1,3] Claw toes increase the slope of the metatarsals. Shortening and fibrosis of the plantar fascia occur. As a result, the pressure under the metatarsal heads increases.[5] Over time, the MTP joints can dislocate, and the plantar pad can migrate distal to the metatarsal heads.[5] As a varus deformity of the hindfoot progresses, the Achilles tendon acts as an invertor.[6] The Achilles tendon shortens over time, leading to a tight calf. This alteration also increases pressure under the metatarsal heads. Moreover, imbalance of intrinsic muscles also promotes the deformity. As the intrinsic flexors are much stronger than the extensors, they overpull them and thus create additional deformation forces.

With further progression of the cavovarus deformity, the talocalcaneal angle typically decreases in the axial and sagittal plane. This results in a more horizontal talar position with a dorsiflexed-like articular position at the tibiotalar joint. The subtalar joint also becomes horizontally aligned, and the talocalcaneal overlap disappears in the sagittal plane. A more horizontal position of the talus may also be a reason why a cavovarus deformity frequently results in impingement at the anteromedial ankle joint. In addition, the calcaneus pitch angle increases on lateral radiographs. The navicular bone turns from a medial to a more superior position relative to the cuboid.[1,4,9] Inclination of the medial metatarsal increases, whereas the fifth metatarsal becomes more horizontal. Due to overloading of the lateral part of the foot, thickening or stress fractures of the fifth metatarsal may occur.[1] More rarely, stress fractures of the cuboid can

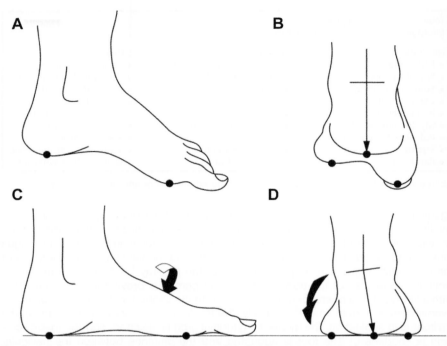

Fig. 3. Forefoot-driven cavovarus deformity. (*A*) The first ray is more plantar flexed in the lateral view. (*B*) Neutral hindfoot alignment (*thin arrow*) of the foot is unloaded. (*C*) When loading, a compensatory varus tilt (*curved arrow*) of the hindfoot occurs. (*D*) Hindfoot alignment (*thin arrow*) shows the varus position (*curved arrow*) of the hindfoot.

also occur.[6] The fibula is slightly posteriorly rotated. In the case of an underlying neurologic disease, the overdrive of the tibialis posterior and peroneus longus muscles lead to a subtalar joint inversion that can be indicated on radiographs by detection of a widened sinus tarsi.[1] As the calcaneus is translated inferiorly and medially beneath the talus, a break in the cyma line is visible on dorsoplantar radiographs.[1] A tripod effect, characterized by weightbearing under the first and fifth metatarsal and the heel, is frequently present.

In a longstanding cavovarus deformity, the lateral structures (eg, lateral ligament complex, peroneus tendons) may become insufficient over time (**Fig. 4**).[4] This can result in anterolateral ankle instability, which is associated with peritalar instability.[12] However, this process is not yet fully understood. In addition, a tilt of the talus in the ankle joint mortise may occur, leading to higher intraarticular medial ankle joint pressure and asymmetric degenerative changes of the tibiotalar joint.[4] Cadaver studies have shown that higher pressure in the anteromedial ankle joint can lead to degenerative changes in the ankle joint even without the presence of lateral ankle instability.[13] In general, the degenerative progression of the medial part of the ankle joint is slower compared with the lateral part because the cartilage and subchondral bone is harder and better resistant to alterations of intraarticular pressure distribution.[4] Medial ankle degeneration also facilitates contracture of the medial soft tissue (eg, deltoid ligament, spring ligament). In longstanding disorders, the initially flexible deformity becomes rigid over time. In the case of a forefoot-driven cavovarus deformity, the flexibility of the hindfoot can be examined using the Coleman block test (**Fig. 5**).[14]

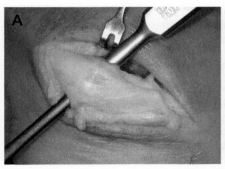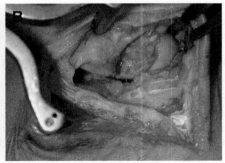

Fig. 4. Operative treatment of a patient suffering of a cavovarus deformity. (*A*) Thickened and scarred peroneal tendons. (*B*) The subtalar joint is spread, and the posterior facet is visible. Subluxation of the talonavicular joint is evident, and the talus is in a more horizontal position.

The effect of a cavovarus deformity on the biomechanics of the foot and ankle is difficult to understand. Abnormalities in the frontal, transversal, and sagittal plane occur, leading to asymmetric force distribution during the gait cycle.[4] To understand the effect of a more plantarflexed first ray, one should be aware that the foot passes a more flexible phase during heelstrike and a more rigid phase while in heel-off. The flexible phase is characterized by relative valgus of the calcaneus, eversion of the subtalar joint, and nonparallelism of the talus and calcaneus.[6,15] In normal feet, the force of the heelstrike can be absorbed during the flexible phase. With further progression of the gait cycle, a relative varus position of the calcaneus occurs.[6] The subtalar joint inverts, and the talus and calcaneus become parallel.[6,15] The foot is stiffer in this position and can act as a lever for heel-off. Increased plantarflexion of the forefoot causes a primary touch of the ground by the first metatarsal. This leads to a compensatory varus heel, a lock of the midfoot, a reduction of the flexible phase, and a decrease in shock absorption.[15,16] While in the heel-off position, a plantarflexed first ray causes a supination of

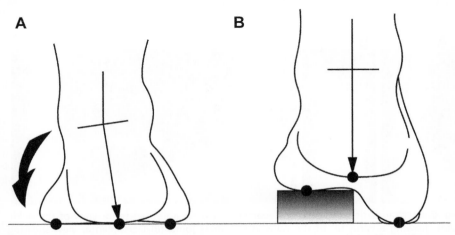

Fig. 5. Coleman block test. (*A*) Forefoot-driven varus (*curved arrow*) hindfoot alignment (*thin arrow*). (*B*) In the case of a flexible hindfoot, the heel is in a neutral position (*thin arrow*) after elevating the lateral part of the forefoot.

the forefoot. Thus, the varus position of the heel increases and the Achilles tendon acts as a supinator. This double effect may further develop the cavovarus deformity. Metatarsalgia and heel pain may occur over time.[6]

HINDFOOT-DRIVEN CAVOVARUS DEFORMITY

Trauma is a frequent reason for hindfoot-driven cavovarus deformity.[1] For example, malunion of pilon fractures with varus angulation of the distal tibial plafond, malunion of talus neck or calcaneus fractures, or longstanding ankle or subtalar joint instability can lead to a varus deformity of the hindfoot (see **Table 1**). To provide a plantigrade position of the foot, a cavus deformity can be developed over time. In feet with hindfoot varus deformity, the talus is frequently found in a dorsiflexion or neutral position (sagittal plane).[17] In the horizontal plane, the talus can either be in a neutral position or externally or internally rotated (**Fig. 6**).[17] In the case of asymmetric ankle osteoarthritis (tilt of the talus >4° in the ankle joint mortise), a defect of the medial distal tibial plafond is often present.[18,19] Additionally, the center of the talus is shifted on anteroposterior radiographs in relation to the tibial axis.[19] Operative reconstruction of the osseous defect of the medial part of the distal tibial plafond is particularly challenging.[19]

Several investigators described a compensatory mechanism of the subtalar joint in the case of a varus hindfoot deformity.[20–24] The ability of the subtalar joint to compensate for deformities above or through the ankle joint can be explained when considering the orientation and geometry of the posterior facet of the calcaneus. Manter[25] compared the posterior facet of a right calcaneus with a right-handed screw. If supramalleolar deformities occur, a healthy subtalar joint theoretically has the possibility to tilt in the opposite direction, compensating for the deformity. Thus, the hindfoot is well-balanced. Compensation of the subtalar joint has recently been found in up to 53% of varus ankle osteoarthritis cases.[24] This study included 226 subjects with ankle osteoarthritis (varus, valgus, and neutral hindfoot alignment).[24]

With the introduction of weightbearing computed tomography (CT) scans, a more detailed analysis of the hindfoot became possible.[26] The talocalcaneal relationship in the case of varus ankle osteoarthritis was studied by several investigators to better understand compensation possibilities for ankle joint deformities on the level of the

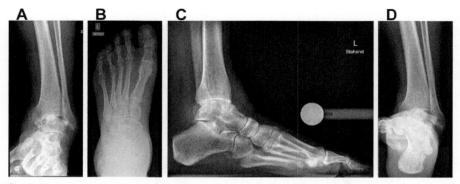

Fig. 6. Posttraumatic varus ankle osteoarthritis. (*A*) An anteroposterior view of the ankle joint showing a varus tilt of the talus in the ankle joint. (*B*) Dorsoplantar view showing medial deviation of the navicular bone and slight pronation of the midfoot and forefoot. (*C*) Lateral view showing distinct degenerative changes of the ankle joint. (*D*) Hindfoot alignment view showing a varus tilt of the hindfoot.

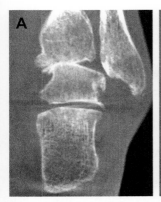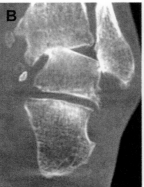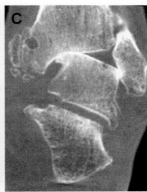

Fig. 7. Assessment of the same patient using weightbearing CT scans showing the screw-shape morphology of the posterior facet of the subtalar joint. (*A*) The posterior part of the posterior facet of the subtalar joint is in a neutral position. (*B*) A slight varus configuration is evident at the middle part of the posterior facet. (*C*) The anterior part of the posterior facet is almost parallel to the talar dome (varus position).

subtalar joint.[22–24,27] The subtalar joint orientation in the coronal plane changes from a varus inclination (posterior) to a more valgus inclination in the anterior part (screw shape anatomy; **Fig. 7**).[23] Overall, a more valgus inclination on the level of the subtalar joint was found in the case of a varus ankle deformity.[22] This finding supports the idea of a compensatory mechanism of the subtalar joint for deformities above the ankle joint.[22] However, it is still questionable to what extent the subtalar joint can compensate for deformities above the ankle joint. In addition, the influence of the subtalar joint shape (eg, a dome-shape or a flat-shape posterior facet) on this compensatory mechanism is not yet fully understood.

A more recent study investigated the talar orientation in the sagittal plane using weightbearing CT scans.[28] In varus ankle osteoarthritis, an abnormal internal rotation of the talus was frequently found. This finding correlated with the stage of ankle osteoarthritis. Higher stages showed a more pronounced internal rotation of the talus compared with lower stages of varus ankle osteoarthritis.

SUMMARY

The cause of cavovarus deformity is various. Based on pathomechanics, one can divide deformities into either forefoot-driven or hindfoot-driven. Alteration of pressure distribution throughout the foot and ankle occurs over time, leading to lateral ankle joint instability and medial ankle osteoarthritis. Increased pressure on bony prominences (eg, metatarsals) is associated with foot pain that is independent of the cause of the cavovarus deformity.[29] This is particularly of interest in patients with metabolic diseases (eg, diabetes mellitus) because increased foot pressure is associated with a higher incidence of chronic ulcerations.[30] In the case of a posttraumatic hindfoot-driven cavovarus deformity, more research is needed to better understand the ability of the subtalar joint to compensate for varus deformities on or above the ankle joint.

ACKNOWLEDGMENTS

We would like to thank Beat Hintermann, MD, and Alexej Barg, MD, for their clinical insights. In addition, we would like to thank Nathan P. Davidson, BS, for making the figures.

REFERENCES

1. Apostle KL, Sangeorzan BJ. Anatomy of the varus foot and ankle. Foot Ankle Clin 2012;17(1):1–11.
2. Maynou C, Szymanski C, Thiounn A. The adult cavus foot. EFORT Open Rev 2017;2(5):221–9.
3. Nogueira MP, Farcetta F, Zuccon A. Cavus foot. Foot Ankle Clin 2015;20(4): 645–56.
4. Klammer G, Benninger E, Espinosa N. The varus ankle and instability. Foot Ankle Clin 2012;17(1):57–82.
5. Younger AS, Hansen ST Jr. Adult cavovarus foot. J Am Acad Orthop Surg 2005; 13(5):302–15.
6. Deben SE, Pomeroy GC. Subtle cavus foot: diagnosis and management. J Am Acad Orthop Surg 2014;22(8):512–20.
7. Faldini C, Traina F, Nanni M, et al. Surgical treatment of cavus foot in Charcot-Marie-tooth disease: a review of twenty-four cases: AAOS exhibit selection. J Bone Joint Surg Am 2015;97(6):e30.
8. Ippolito E. Update on pathologic anatomy of clubfoot. J Pediatr Orthop B 1995; 4(1):17–24.
9. Aminian A, Sangeorzan BJ. The anatomy of cavus foot deformity. Foot Ankle Clin 2008;13(2):191–8, v.
10. Manoli A 2nd, Graham B. The subtle cavus foot, "the underpronator". Foot Ankle Int 2005;26(3):256–63.
11. Weinberg MW, Krahenbuhl N, Davidson NP, et al. Isolated avulsion fracture of the first metatarsal base at the peroneus longus tendon attachment: a case report. Skeletal Radiol 2018;47(5):743–6.
12. Hintermann B, Knupp M, Barg A. Peritalar instability. Foot Ankle Int 2012;33(5): 450–4.
13. Krause F, Windolf M, Schwieger K, et al. Ankle joint pressure in pes cavovarus. J Bone Joint Surg Br 2007;89(12):1660–5.
14. Coleman SS, Chesnut WJ. A simple test for hindfoot flexibility in the cavovarus foot. Clin Orthop Relat Res 1977;(123):60–2.
15. Schwend RM, Drennan JC. Cavus foot deformity in children. J Am Acad Orthop Surg 2003;11(3):201–11.
16. Chilvers M, Manoli A 2nd. The subtle cavus foot and association with ankle instability and lateral foot overload. Foot Ankle Clin 2008;13(2):315–24, vii.
17. Nosewicz TL, Knupp M, Bolliger L, et al. Radiological morphology of peritalar instability in varus and valgus tilted ankles. Foot Ankle Int 2014;35(5):453–62.
18. Cox JS, Hewes TF. "Normal" talar tilt angle. Clin Orthop Relat Res 1979;140: 37–41.
19. Hintermann B, Ruiz R, Barg A. Novel double osteotomy technique of distal tibia for correction of asymmetric varus osteoarthritic ankle. Foot Ankle Int 2017; 38(9):970–81.
20. Hayashi K, Tanaka Y, Kumai T, et al. Correlation of compensatory alignment of the subtalar joint to the progression of primary osteoarthritis of the ankle. Foot Ankle Int 2008;29(4):400–6.
21. Krahenbuhl N, Horn-Lang T, Hintermann B, et al. The subtalar joint: a complex mechanism. EFORT Open Rev 2017;2(7):309–16.
22. Krahenbuhl N, Siegler L, Deforth M, et al. Subtalar joint alignment in ankle osteoarthritis. Foot Ankle Surg 2017. [Epub ahead of print].

23. Krahenbuhl N, Tschuck M, Bolliger L, et al. Orientation of the subtalar joint: measurement and reliability using weightbearing CT scans. Foot Ankle Int 2016;37(1):109–14.
24. Wang B, Saltzman CL, Chalayon O, et al. Does the subtalar joint compensate for ankle malalignment in end-stage ankle arthritis? Clin Orthop Relat Res 2015; 473(1):318–25.
25. Manter JT. Movements of the subtalar and trensverse tarsal joints. Anat Rec 1941;80:397.
26. Barg A, Bailey T, Richter M, et al. Weightbearing computed tomography of the foot and ankle: emerging technology topical review. Foot Ankle Int 2018;39(3): 376–86.
27. Burssens A, Peeters J, Buedts K, et al. Measuring hindfoot alignment in weight bearing CT: a novel clinical relevant measurement method. Foot Ankle Surg 2016;22(4):233–8.
28. Kim JB, Yi Y, Kim JY, et al. Weight-bearing computed tomography findings in varus ankle osteoarthritis: abnormal internal rotation of the talus in the axial plane. Skeletal Radiol 2017;46(8):1071–80.
29. Burns J, Crosbie J, Hunt A, et al. The effect of pes cavus on foot pain and plantar pressure. Clin Biomech (Bristol, Avon) 2005;20(9):877–82.
30. Ledoux WR, Shofer JB, Ahroni JH, et al. Biomechanical differences among pes cavus, neutrally aligned, and pes planus feet in subjects with diabetes. Foot Ankle Int 2003;24(11):845–50.

Clinical Examination and Radiographic Assessment of the Cavus Foot

Craig C. Akoh, MD[a],*, Phinit Phisitkul, MD[b]

KEYWORDS

- Cavus • Cavovarus • Meary angle • Radiograph • Clinical examination

KEY POINTS

- The clinical evaluation of the cavus foot should determine whether the deformity is forefoot-driven or hindfoot-driven.
- Gait analysis and shoe wear patterns are the first steps in a thorough examination.
- Lateral column overloading manifests with callosities and pain along the plantar foot.
- Plain radiographic assessment is critical for the assessment of the cavus foot. A variety of radiographic measurements can confirm the clinical diagnosis.
- Advanced imaging can assess for tarsal coalitions and soft tissue pathologies.

CLINICAL EXAMINATION

The purpose of the clinical examination is to detect subtle cavus or cavovarus deformity, assess the severity and type of deformity, differentiate between an idiopathic versus secondary etiologies of cavus foot deformity, and evaluate for other associated abnormalities. An individual with cavus foot deformity can present with a wide range of clinical signs and symptoms depending on the severity of the underlying deformity. The common clinical finding of the cavus foot is a high plantar arch.[1,2] Patients with cavus deformities often present around puberty, as muscle imbalances and changes in bony anatomy become more pronounced. These patients typically present with lateral foot pain or gait disturbances.[3] In addition, frequent falls can occur due to muscle imbalances and lateral ankle instability.[4] It is important to obtain a thorough family

Disclosure Statement: The authors report the following potential conflicts of interest or sources of funding: P. Phisitkul is a paid consultant for Arthrex and Restor 3D, receives royalties from Arthrex, and has stock/stock options in First Ray and Mortise Medical. Full ICMJE author disclosure forms are available for this article online, as supplementary material.

[a] Department of Orthopedics and Rehabilitation, University of Wisconsin School of Medicine and Public Health Madison, 600 Highland Avenue, Room 6220, Madison, WI 53705-2281, USA;
[b] Tri-State Specialists, LLP, 2730 Pierce Street, Suite 300, Sioux City, IA 51104, USA
* Corresponding author.
E-mail address: ccakoh@gmail.com

history because family members with similar symptoms may signify a genetic etiology for the cavus foot deformity.

Musculoskeletal Examination

The clinical examination of the cavus foot should begin with a gait analysis. It is important to delineate the foot position during the various phases of the gait cycle. Proper balance of the foot is achieved by establishing a balanced tripod. The centers of pressure should be within the 3 points of contact along the plantar surface of the foot. These points include the plantar heel, the medial forefoot, and the lateral forefoot. Patients with cavus feet often have an underlying muscle imbalance that leads to an unbalanced tripod, pressure overloading, and subsequent gait alteration. During heel strike, the cavus foot is unable to unlock the Chopart joint, leading to a rigid midfoot and lack of proper stress distribution.[5] During toe-off, midfoot cavus is significantly increased due to the hyperextended metatarsophalangeal (MTP) joint and increased windlass effect on the plantar fascia.[6] Rotational alignment should be assessed both during gait by measuring the foot progression angle and in the prone position by measuring the transmalleolar axis. The tibia normally has 15° of external rotation, which can be increased in cavus foot deformities.[7]

Visual inspection of both feet is paramount in the thorough evaluation of the cavus foot. The patient should have the feet shoulder-width apart. In addition, the medial border of both feet should be parallel with each other to negate any differences in lower extremity rotation.[8] Subtle limb length discrepancy or asymmetric foot size can be a result of residual clubfoot or poliomyelitis. Posteromedial incisions can indicate previous surgically treated clubfoot deformities. Previous burns or scars, as well as muscle atrophy, could represent a traumatic etiology or missed compartment syndrome. Abnormal shoe wear pattern of the lateral midfoot region can be the first sign that a patient has a cavus foot deformity.

During inspection, the clinician should determine whether the cavus foot is forefoot-driven, hindfoot-driven, or mixed.[9] Visualization of the foot from the front allows for the assessment of forefoot-driven cavus foot deformity. Forefoot-driven cavus is a result of a plantarflexed and pronated first ray in relation to the midfoot. There is a compensatory flexible hindfoot varus deformity to improve stress distribution along the plantar foot. Patients with an equinus contracture can exacerbate the plantarflexion deformity of the first ray secondary to the unopposed peroneus longus tendon.[10] Hindfoot varus can also may manifest as a "peek-a-boo" heel. First described by Manoli and colleagues,[11,12] the "peek-a-boo" heel occurs when the medial heel pad is visible when viewing the anterior foot (**Fig. 1**). False-positive "peek-a-boo" heel can occur with a large heel pad, external tibial torsion, metatarsus adductus, and inability to place feet together in obese patients with thigh impingement.[1,8] Confirmation of a "peek-a-boo" heel should be made with the posterior inspection of the heel. The clinician also may notice a prominent extensor digitorum brevis muscle along the dorsolateral aspect of the foot as a result of the varus hindfoot alignment.[8] Lesser toe deformities, such as claw toeing, can be present in patients with underlying neurologic etiologies for pes cavus. Claw toe is caused by weak intrinsic foot muscles and unopposed long toe extensor tendons. This results in the hyperextension of the MTP joint and subsequent toe clawing.[13] Proximal migration of the plantar heel pad can make the lesser metatarsal heads more prominent. Metatarsus adductus of the forefoot also may be present and is diagnosed when the heel bisector line crosses lateral to the second toe. Patients with residual clubfoot deformities also may have a dorsally subluxed navicular bone and dorsal bunion of the great toe.[14,15] The inspection of the plantar aspect of the foot can reveal callosities under the base of the fifth

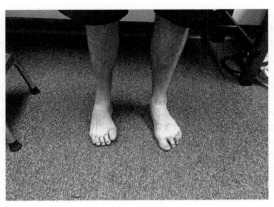

Fig. 1. Peek-a-boo heel.

metatarsal and under the first metatarsal head as a result of uneven stress distribution of the cavus foot. A tight medial longitudinal plantar fascia with or without local tenderness also may be appreciated.

Posterior evaluation of the cavus foot can assess for hindfoot-driven pes cavus. Hindfoot-driven pes cavus is much rarer than forefoot-driven pes cavus. Normally, the heel should be lateral to the midline of the calf due to the 5° valgus position of the calcaneus. When the hindfoot is in varus, the heel becomes positioned medial to the midline of the calf and the lateral midfoot becomes prominent. Patients with hindfoot-driven deformity have a markedly vertical calcaneus due to a weak gastrocnemius-soleus complex. Several neurologic conditions are associated with calcaneocavus deformity, including poliomyelitis, iatrogenic weakness after cerebral palsy treatment, spinal dysraphism, and intraspinal etiologies.[9] The Coleman block test is performed to confirm whether the cavus deformity is forefoot-driven or hindfoot-driven[16] (**Fig. 2**) This test is performed by placing a 1-inch block under the lateral foot, allowing the first ray to be unsupported. This eliminates the forefoot pronation and compensatory hindfoot varus. In a forefoot-driven deformity, the hindfoot will correct to neutral or valgus when visualized from the rear. A rigid hindfoot-driven deformity will not correct with the Coleman block test, necessitating further investigation for tarsal coalition, subtalar arthritis, or spasticity. Other conditions that can mimic a

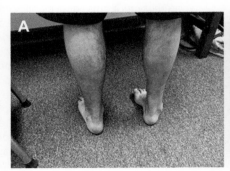
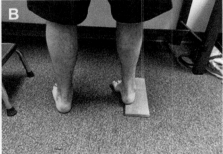

Fig. 2. Hindfoot examination. (*A*) Hindfoot from posterior before posting and (*B*) partial correction of varus heel with Coleman block testing.

cavus foot position due to protective supination include painful plantar fasciitis, sesamoiditis, and stress fractures.[8]

Palpation of the foot and ankle should be performed with the patient in the seated position. Careful examination can reveal areas of overloading associated with the cavus foot. The lateral column is the most common site of pain.[17] Specifically, palpating the base of the fourth and fifth metatarsals can reveal pain from a stress fracture or stress reaction.[18,19] A history of nonhealing proximal fractures of the lateral metatarsal bones also should warrant workup for metatarsal adductus and cavus alignment.[20] Increased plantarflexion of the first ray can cause pain along the plantar MTP joint and sesamoiditis of the great toe. Palpation along the medial plantar fascia can reveal pain or stiffness. Retro-fibular pain at the lateral malleolus can be due to peroneal tendon pathology. On clinical examination, retro-fibular pain can be elicited by the activation of peroneal muscles. Anteromedial ankle pain can reveal soft tissue impingement or intra-articular pathology. Lateral collateral ligament incompetency can be detected by palpating the anterior talofibular ligament and calcaneofibular ligaments. A ligamentous examination, including the anterior drawer and talar tilt test should be performed if ankle instability is suspected.[4]

Evaluation of range of motion throughout the various joints within the foot and ankle can facilitate in the appropriate management of pes cavus. In the seated position, both active and passive ankle range of motion should be assessed. The inability to dorsiflex the ankle past neutral is commonly due to an equinus contracture. The Silfverskiold test can be used to differentiate between an isolated gastrocnemius and Achilles contracture.[21,22] The Silfverskiold test is performed with both examiner's hands on the foot (Fig. 3). One hand is placed at the level of the subtalar joint and the other hand is placed at the midfoot to stabilize the talonavicular joint during ankle dorsiflexion. The clinician then passively dorsiflexes the ankle both with the knee fully extended

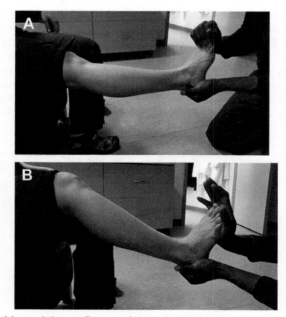

Fig. 3. Silfverskiold test. (*A*) Dorsiflexion of the ankle with the knee in full extension and (*B*) dorsiflexion of the ankle with the knee in flexion.

and the knee at 90° of flexion to relax the gastrocnemius muscle. The inability to dorsi-flex the ankle to neutral with the knee extended denotes an isolated gastrocnemius contracture. The inability to dorsiflex the ankle with the knee partially flexed denotes a combined gastrocnemius-soleus contracture. Limited ankle dorsiflexion also can be due to anteromedial ankle impingement from a dorsiflexed talus within the ankle mortis in patients with residual clubfoot. Subtalar arthritis can be ruled out with a sup-ple hindfoot examination.[23] The patient should perform single and double-legged heel raises to assess the dynamic flexibility of the subtalar joint. The ability of the subtalar joint to evert when the heel is on the ground and invert during heel raises decreases the likelihood of hindfoot arthritis. The Kelikian test can be used to assess the flexibility of claw toe deformity at the MTP joint.[3] Passive hyperextension of the lesser metatarsal heads tightens the plantar fascia and can correct a flexible claw toe deformity. If the claw toe deformity does not correct, then it is rigid. In general, passively correctable deformities are amendable to tendon transfers, whereas rigid deformities require osteotomy or salvage procedures.

Neurologic Examination

One of the key components in a thorough examination for patients with cavus foot de-formities is the neurologic examination. The neurologic examination can clue a clini-cian on a potential systemic peripheral neuropathy or central nervous system etiology for the foot deformity. A complete upper and lower motor neurologic exami-nation includes inspection, reflex testing, and upper motor neuron testing. Patients with severe bilateral cavus feet and clawing should undergo electromyogram testing to screen for peripheral nerve disorders such as Charcot-Marie-Tooth (CMT) disease. One study found that the incidence of CMT in patients with bilateral cavus foot was 78%.[24] In addition, a positive family history increases the incidence of CMT in patients with bilateral cavus to 91%. Patients with CMT often have intrinsic wasting, which is most noticeable in the first dorsal interossei muscle of the hand. Patients with arthrog-ryposis can have contractures involving their upper extremities. Abnormal reflexes and upper motor neuron signs (ie, Babinski test and Hoffman test) can signify a central ner-vous system etiology. Patients with Friedreich ataxia present with progressive cavus deformity in the second decade of life. The clinical triad for Friedreich ataxia includes ataxia, positive Babinski, and areflexia.[5] Patients with cerebral palsy can develop equinovarus foot deformity with underlying tibialis anterior spasticity.[5] Finally, a spine examination should be performed to assess for midline abnormalities, such as hair tuft, skin dimple, or skin patch. These midline abnormalities could signify an underlying spinal dysraphism and spinal imaging should be obtained. Asymmetric or rapidly pro-gressing cavus deformities also warrant spinal imaging to rule out intraspinal pathol-ogies such as an intraspinal tumor or tethered cord.

A complete motor examination also should accompany a neurologic examination. Assessment of muscle power should be graded using the Medical Research Council (MRC) grading system. The MRC system grades muscle strength from 1 to 5 and is as follows: grade 1: flicker of contraction; grade 2: partial antigravity strength; grade 3: full antigravity strength with full range of motion; grade 4: partial strength against resis-tance; grade 5: full strength against resistance. Often the intrinsic muscles of the foot are affected first in patients with CMT because longer peripheral nerves are pref-erentially affected. Patients with CMT with weak tibialis anterior musculature can lead to unopposed plantarflexion of the first ray by the peroneus longus and forefoot-driven cavus deformity. Preferential weakness of the peroneal brevis muscle can lead to un-opposed pull of the tibialis posterior muscle, leading to hindfoot varus and in the cavus foot (**Fig. 4**). Gastrocnemius weakness can be seen in patients with poliomyelitis or

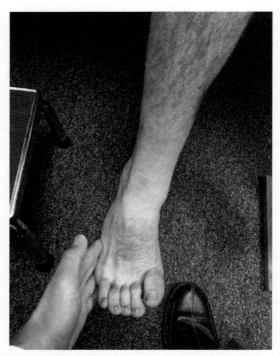

Fig. 4. Peroneus brevis strength testing.

surgically treated patients with cerebral palsy, leading to calcaneovarus and hindfoot-driven deformity. Patients with poliomyelitis may have weakness and limb length discrepancy of the affected extremity without intrinsic foot weakness. Patients with cerebral palsy often have muscle spasticity of the tibialis anterior during gait and rigid lesser toe deformities. Patients with residual clubfoot often present with dynamic supination due to a strong tibialis anterior and weak antagonist muscles.[14,25] Knowing the muscle strength of select tendons can assist with tendon transfer options.

RADIOGRAPHIC ASSESSMENT

Plain radiographic assessment is critical for the assessment of the cavus foot. A variety of radiographic measurements can confirm the clinical diagnosis. The standard plain *weight-bearing* radiographic series includes ankle series (anteroposterior [AP], lateral) and foot series (standing bilateral AP, lateral, and hindfoot) (**Fig. 5**). In general, obtaining the ankle and foot on the same cassette allows for the overall nature of the deformity to be optimally visualized.[26] Rotational deformity is an important aspect of cavus deformity. When assessing the ankle radiographically, attention to the position of the fibula can aid in the assessment of lower extremity rotation. A posteriorly positioned fibula on the lateral plain radiograph is indicative of an externally rotated tibia. A sinus-tarsi see-though sign and double talar dome sign also can indicate external rotation of the ankle joint. Rotational deformity can make obtaining a true lateral of the ankle joint and the talar dome difficult. Internally rotating the leg can assist in obtaining a true lateral of the ankle joint to allow the clinician to assess for arthritic changes at the tibiotalar joint.

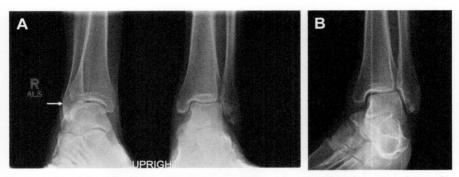

Fig. 5. Ankle plain radiographs. (*A*) Bilateral standing AP ankle (*B*) and mortise plain radiographs. Notice the externally rotated ankle and increased overlap between the lateral malleolus and distal tibia (*white arrow*).

On the standing lateral foot view (**Fig. 6**), it is important to determine the apex of the cavus deformity for surgical planning. Forefoot-driven deformity can be assessed using the Meary angle, which is measured between the long axis of the talus and first metatarsal bone.[27] The normal Meary angle should measure 0 ± 5°, indicating that the first metatarsal is in line with the long axis of the talus. A Meary angle greater than 5° indicates increased plantarflexion of the first metatarsal in relation to the long axis of the talus. The average Meary angle for patients with cavus feet is 18°.[28] Hindfoot-driven deformity is measured by the calcaneal pitch and Hibb angle. The calcaneal pitch is measured using the angle between the horizontal plane of the heel and axis of the heel. Normal value is 22°. A calcaneal pitch greater than 30° is considered to be indicative of a hindfoot-driven cavus deformity.[8] The Hibb angle (calcaneal-first metatarsal angle) is measured between the longitudinal axis of the calcaneus and first metatarsal. Normal is less than 45°. Patients with cavus foot deformities have an angle greater than 90°.[5,23] The lateral talocalcaneal angle can be reduced (<25°) in patients with residual clubfoot deformity, resulting in hindfoot parallelism. The medial-cuneiform height can be used to measure the severity of midfoot cavus. It is the distance between the plantar-most aspect of the distal medial-cuneiform and plantar-most aspect of the distal fifth metatarsal. A measurement greater than 13 mm denotes a cavus foot.[29] The oblique foot view can assess for any stress fractures at metatarsal shafts due to overloading of the lateral column.

The bilateral standing AP foot view can aid in visualizing the coronal alignment of the forefoot (**Fig. 7**). Metatarsus adductus can be seen best with this view. Overlapping of the base of the metatarsals indicates forefoot pronation. In addition, periosteal

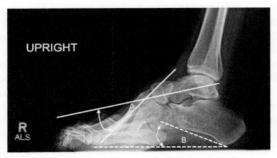

Fig. 6. Lateral foot plain radiograph. Meary angle (angle A) and calcaneal pitch (angle B).

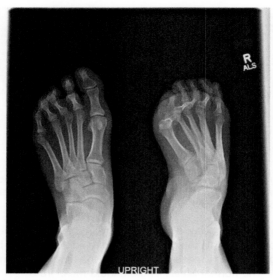

Fig. 7. AP bilateral standing plain radiographs.

reaction and callous formation can indicate stress fractures along the base of the fifth metatarsal or the lesser metatarsal bones. Talocalcaneal overcoverage can be measured from the angle from the perpendicular surfaces of the talar head and navicular.[29,30] An AP talocalcaneal angle greater than 7° indicates forefoot adduction. It is difficult to radiographically diagnose cavus deformities given distorted anatomy and the cumbersome nature of multiple radiographic measures. As a result, tripod index was described by Arunakul and colleagues[29] a simplified additive measurement for compensatory deformities at the foot. On the standing AP view, a heel marker is placed along the posterior heel. The angles measured include (1) a lateral angle from the center of the hemispherical marker, the lateral fifth metatarsal bone, and the medial sesamoid, and (2) a medial angle is measured from the center hemispherical marker to the medial sesamoid and the center of the talar head (**Fig. 8**). The tripod index is the ratio between the medial angle/lateral angles × 100. A negative tripod index less than −39% denotes a cavus foot, denoting talonavicular overcoverage. The tripod index has been found to be highly sensitive and specific for diagnosing cavus deformities.[31]

The standing hindfoot view was first described by Cobey[32] and later modified by Saltzman and el-Khoury.[33] To obtain the modified hindfoot view, the patient stands on a radiolucent platform with the feet internally rotated to be parallel with each other. The radiograph cassette is then held 20° from vertical. The radiographic beam is aimed perpendicular to the cassette (20° caudal from horizontal) and centered between both ankles. The final radiographic image should contain the distal tibia to the calcaneus. Although very reliable, some investigators are concerned that this modified hindfoot view does not represent the true coronal calcaneus axis and is highly variable depending on leg rotation.[34] Reilingh and colleagues described[35] the long axial view, which is performed with the patient in a bilateral weight-bearing stance. The cassette is placed on the plantar surface of the foot and the radiograph beam is aimed 45° caudal from the floor. They found that the long axial view had improved interobserver reliability when compared with the modified hindfoot view.

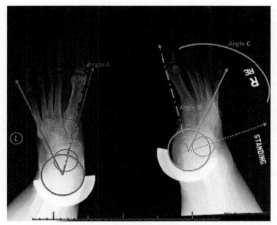

Fig. 8. Tripod index. Tripod index for the left normal foot = (a/b × 100) = 5/34 × 100 = 14.7%. The Tripod index for the right cavovarus foot is (c/d × 100) = −76/39 × 100 = −194.9%.

Advanced imaging can also assist in diagnosing pathology associated with pes cavus. The weight-bearing computed tomography (CT) scan can assess for subtalar coalitions or arthritis in patients with rigid hindfoot deformity. If rotational malalignment is suspected clinically, then lower extremity CT scans can assess for external tibial torsion. Knupp and colleagues[36] published a comparative study of combined single-photon emission computed tomography (SPECT/CT) technique versus conventional CT imaging for ankle loading in hindfoot malalignment. They found that increased positron activity was seen at the medial ankle in patients with varus hindfoot alignment. The increase in positron activity correlated with the location of plain radiograph osteoarthritis. MRI can be used to assess for soft tissue pathology such as peroneal tendinitis, tears, osteochondral lesions, and fibrous tarsal coalitions. Digital dynamic pedobarography can be used to assess pathologic pressure along the plantar foot during standing and gait.[37] Surgical intervention can lead to increased foot contact area and decreased overloading of the lateral midfoot.[38,39]

In addition, various studies have shown mild correlation with radiographic correction of the Meary angle and Hibbs angle with improved foot contact pressures.[39,40]

SUMMARY

The clinical evaluation of the cavus foot should determine whether the deformity is forefoot-driven or hindfoot-driven. Gait analysis and shoe wear patterns are the first steps in a thorough examination. Inspection of both feet is important to assess the severity and symmetry of the deformities. Lateral column overloading manifests with callosities and pain along the plantar foot. Muscle strength and imbalances should be assessed to determine the etiology and treatment. Last, individuals with rapidly progressing cavus deformities or asymmetry should undergo neurologic testing and spine imaging.

REFERENCES

1. Manoli A 2nd, Graham B. The subtle cavus foot, "the underpronator". Foot Ankle Int 2005;26(3):256–63.

2. Holmes JR, Hansen ST Jr. Foot and ankle manifestations of Charcot-Marie-Tooth disease. Foot Ankle 1993;14(8):476–86.
3. Nogueira MP, Farcetta F, Zuccon A. Cavus foot. Foot Ankle Clin 2015;20(4): 645–56.
4. Chilvers M, Manoli A 2nd. The subtle cavus foot and association with ankle instability and lateral foot overload. Foot Ankle Clin 2008;13(2):315–24, vii.
5. Schwend RM, Drennan JC. Cavus foot deformity in children. J Am Acad Orthop Surg 2003;11(3):201–11.
6. Sabir M, Lyttle D. Pathogenesis of pes cavus in Charcot-Marie-Tooth disease. Clin Orthop Relat Res 1983;(175):173–8.
7. Hansen ST. The cavovarus/supinated foot deformity and external tibial torsion: the role of the posterior tibial tendon. Foot Ankle Clin 2008;13(2):325–8, viii.
8. Abbasian A, Pomeroy G. The idiopathic cavus foot-not so subtle after all. Foot Ankle Clin 2013;18(4):629–42.
9. Japas LM. Surgical treatment of pes cavus by tarsal V-osteotomy. Preliminary report. J Bone Joint Surg Am 1968;50(5):927–44.
10. Silver RL, de la Garza J, Rang M. The myth of muscle balance. A study of relative strengths and excursions of normal muscles about the foot and ankle. J Bone Joint Surg Br 1985;67(3):432–7.
11. Beals TC, Manoli A. The peek-a-boo heel sign in the evaluation of hindfoot varus. Foot 1996;6:205–6.
12. Manoli A 2nd, Smith DG, Hansen ST Jr. Scarred muscle excision for the treatment of established ischemic contracture of the lower extremity. Clin Orthop Relat Res 1993;(292):309–14.
13. Myerson MS, Shereff MJ. The pathological anatomy of claw and hammer toes. J Bone Joint Surg Am 1989;71(1):45–9.
14. Uglow MG, Kurup HV. Residual clubfoot in children. Foot Ankle Clin 2010;15(2): 245–64.
15. Ward CM, Dolan LA, Bennett DL, et al. Long-term results of reconstruction for treatment of a flexible cavovarus foot in Charcot-Marie-Tooth disease. J Bone Joint Surg Am 2008;90(12):2631–42.
16. Coleman SS, Chesnut WJ. A simple test for hindfoot flexibility in the cavovarus foot. Clin Orthop Relat Res 1977;(123):60–2.
17. Krause FG, Guyton GP. Pes cavus. In: Coughlin MJ, SC, editors. Mann's surgery of the foot and ankle. 9th edition. Philadelphia: Elsevier Inc; 2014. p. 1361–82.
18. Saxena A, Krisdakumtorn T, Erickson S. Proximal fourth metatarsal injuries in athletes: similarity to proximal fifth metatarsal injury. Foot Ankle Int 2001;22(7):603–8.
19. Rongstad KM, Tueting J, Rongstad M, et al. Fourth metatarsal base stress fractures in athletes: a case series. Foot Ankle Int 2013;34(7):962–8.
20. O'Malley M, DeSandis B, Allen A, et al. Operative treatment of fifth metatarsal Jones fractures (zones II and III) in the NBA. Foot Ankle Int 2016;37(5):488–500.
21. Silfverskiöld N. Reduction of the uncrossed two-joints muscles of the leg to one-joint muscles in spastic conditions. Acta Chir Scand 1924;56:315–30.
22. DiGiovanni CW, Kuo R, Tejwani N, et al. Isolated gastrocnemius tightness. J Bone Joint Surg Am 2002;84-a(6):962–70.
23. Marks RM. Midfoot and forefoot issues cavovarus foot: assessment and treatment issues. Foot Ankle Clin 2008;13(2):229–41, vi.
24. Nagai MK, Chan G, Guille JT, et al. Prevalence of Charcot-Marie-Tooth disease in patients who have bilateral cavovarus feet. J Pediatr Orthop 2006;26(4):438–43.

25. Holt JB, Oji DE, Yack HJ, et al. Long-term results of tibialis anterior tendon transfer for relapsed idiopathic clubfoot treated with the Ponseti method: a follow-up of thirty-seven to fifty-five years. J Bone Joint Surg Am 2015;97(1):47–55.
26. Perera AG, Guha A. Clinical and radiographic evaluation of the cavus foot: surgical implications. In: Kadakia A, editor. Innovations in the cavus foot deformity, an issue of foot and ankle clinics. 1st edition. Philadelphia: Elsevier; 2013. p. 619–88.
27. Meary R. On the measurement of the angle between the talus and the first metatarsal. Rev Chir Orthop 1967;53:389–91.
28. Alexander IJ, Johnson KA. Assessment and management of pes cavus in Charcot-Marie-Tooth disease. Clin Orthop Relat Res 1989;(246):273–81.
29. Arunakul M, Amendola A, Gao Y, et al. Tripod index: a new radiographic parameter assessing foot alignment. Foot Ankle Int 2013;34(10):1411–20.
30. Sangeorzan BJ, Mosca V, Hansen ST Jr. Effect of calcaneal lengthening on relationships among the hindfoot, midfoot, and forefoot. Foot Ankle 1993;14(3): 136–41.
31. Arunakul M, Amendola A, Gao Y, et al. Tripod Index: diagnostic accuracy in symptomatic flatfoot and cavovarus foot: part 2. Iowa Orthop J 2013;33:47–53.
32. Cobey JC. Posterior roentgenogram of the foot. Clin Orthop Relat Res 1976;(118): 202–7.
33. Saltzman CL, el-Khoury GY. The hindfoot alignment view. Foot Ankle Int 1995; 16(9):572–6.
34. Johnson JE, Lamdan R, Granberry WF, et al. Hindfoot coronal alignment: a modified radiographic method. Foot Ankle Int 1999;20(12):818–25.
35. Reilingh ML, Beimers L, Tuijthof GJ, et al. Measuring hindfoot alignment radiographically: the long axial view is more reliable than the hindfoot alignment view. Skeletal Radiol 2010;39(11):1103–8.
36. Knupp M, Pagenstert GI, Barg A, et al. SPECT-CT compared with conventional imaging modalities for the assessment of the varus and valgus malaligned hindfoot. J Orthop Res 2009;27(11):1461–6.
37. Fernandez-Seguin LM, Diaz Mancha JA, Sanchez Rodriguez R, et al. Comparison of plantar pressures and contact area between normal and cavus foot. Gait Posture 2014;39(2):789–92.
38. Chan G, Sampath J, Miller F, et al. The role of the dynamic pedobarograph in assessing treatment of cavovarus feet in children with Charcot-Marie-Tooth disease. J Pediatr Orthop 2007;27(5):510–6.
39. Erickson S, Hosseinzadeh P, Iwinski HJ, et al. Dynamic pedobarography and radiographic evaluation of surgically treated cavovarus foot deformity in children with Charcot-Marie-Tooth disease. J Pediatr Orthop B 2015;24(4):336–40.
40. Thometz JG, Liu XC, Tassone JC, et al. Correlation of foot radiographs with foot function as analyzed by plantar pressure distribution. J Pediatr Orthop 2005; 25(2):249–52.

Neurologic Disorders and Cavovarus Deformity

Julie A. Neumann, MD*, Florian Nickisch, MD

KEYWORDS

- Cavovarus • Charcot-Marie tooth disease • Neuropathy • Foot

KEY POINTS

- A cavovarus deformity results from muscular imbalances of the foot. Specifically, it can be driven by plantarflexion of the first ray (cavus), which results in inversion of the calcaneus/hindfoot (varus).
- History, physical examination, and imaging help determine appropriate treatment, as the deformity can be flexible or rigid and can present in children or adults.
- Charcot-Marie-Tooth (CMT) disease is the most common inherited neuropathy with approximately 50 genetic subtypes and is a common cause of cavovarus foot deformity.
- Treatment should be individualized and should focus on alleviating symptoms and restoring alignment of the forefoot and hindfoot to obtain and plantigrade foot.
- Non-operative management consists of shoe modifications, physical therapy, orthotics, ankle braces, ankle foot orthosis, and night splints. Operative treatment centers around subtalar joint mobility and consists of soft tissue releases, tendon transfers, osteotomies, arthrodesis, and repair or reconstruction of lateral ankle ligaments and peroneal tendons.

INTRODUCTION

A cavus deformity results from imbalance of muscular forces, specifically when the first ray is plantarflexed in comparison with the hindfoot.[1,2] Plantarflexion of the first ray secondary to weak anterior tibialis and a strong peroneus longus drives the calcaneus into inversion, which gives the varus component to the deformity.[1,2] In other words, an inverted calcaneus is a compensatory mechanism for forefoot equinus and valgus.[1] These 2 deformities together comprise a "cavovarus" foot deformity.[1] The cavovarus deformity is then magnified in the setting of a weak peroneus brevis and strong posterior tibialis.[2] The cavus portion of the deformity is often the consequence of progressive muscle imbalance and results in changes to the ankle, hindfoot, midfoot, and forefoot.[1,2] There are several etiologies of the cavovarus foot deformity

Disclosure Statement: The authors have nothing to disclose.
University of Utah Orthopaedic Department, University Orthopaedic Center, 590 Wakara Way, Salt Lake City, UT 84108, USA
* Corresponding author.
E-mail address: Julie.Neumann.MD@gmail.com

including the following: congenital (hereditary motor and sensory neuropathies, club-foot), neurologic (spinal cord lesions, poliomyelitis, amyotrophic lateral sclerosis commonly known as Lou Gehrig's disease, Friedreich's ataxia, Huntington's chorea, cerebral palsy, and stroke or other cerebral injury), post-traumatic (talar neck injuries), and idiopathic, to name a few.[1,2]

CHARCOT-MARIE-TOOTH DISEASE

One of the most common causes of a cavovarus foot deformity is Charcot-Marie-Tooth (CMT) disease. Charcot-Marie-Tooth disease is the most common inherited neuropathy and is estimated to affect 37/100,000 people.[1,3,4] Charcot-Marie-Tooth disease was originally described in 1884 by Friedrich Schultze.[3] Then, in 1886, a French man Jean-Martin Charcot and his student Pierre Marie coined the term "peroneal muscular atrophy."[5] The same year, in London, Howard Henry Tooth described "The peroneal type of progressive muscular atrophy."[6]

Charcot-Marie-Tooth disease is a hereditary motor and sensory neuropathy and there are approximately 50 genetic subtypes that fall under the catch-all title of CMT.[1,3] Physicians should be aware of the different genetics types of CMT, as the risk of progression and rate of deformity is not the same for various mutations.[3] The most common subgroups are type 1 (two-thirds of patients with CMT) and type 2 (one-third of patients with CMT).[3] The myelin surrounding nerves is abnormal in type 1, thus an electromyogram shows slowing.[3] Charcot-Marie-Tooth type 2 is characterized by abnormal axon function, thus the electromyogram shows normal speed of impulse transfer with decreased magnitude of impulse.[3] Type 3 is Dejerine-Sottas disease, which is severe in clinical manifestation.[2,3] Most commonly CMT is inherited in an autosomal dominant pattern, but it can also be autosomal recessive, or X-linked.[2,3] In CMT type 1A the defect is on chromosome 17 and is most commonly a duplication of a portion of the PMP22 gene.[3,4] Contrarily the gene defect for CMT type 1B is on chromosome 1, and in CMT type 2 it is on chromosomes 1 and 3.[3]

Distal muscle wasting is a characteristic of CMT and often results in foot deformity.[3] Patients with CMT are more likely to have foot deformity than deformity of the hands.[7] Often, these foot deformities are multiplanar and the most common deformity is cavovarus.[1,7] The exception is that type 2 CMT actually has a higher incidence of planovalgus deformity (55%) versus cavovarus deformity (36%).[8] This is similar with cerebral palsy because the deformity depends on which motor cortex is involved, but is estimated to be planovalgus (66%) versus cavovarus (34%).[9]

To date, there are no large studies on the natural history of patients with CMT.[3] However, CMT often progresses, which must be considered when devising a treatment strategy.[3] As with any cavovarus foot deformity, treatment of the deformity associated with CMT is based on the underlying etiology, age of the patient, as well as both the static and dynamic physical examination.[1] In addition, many patients with CMT have atypical bone shapes, as CMT often manifests in children.[3]

The typical order of denervation associated with CMT is the tibial nerve, which affects the intrinsic muscles leading to plantar wasting, contractures, and fibrosis.[1,2] Intrinsic muscle wasting ultimately elevates the longitudinal arch and shortens the foot, because the long flexors and extensors overpower the lumbrical and interossei muscles.[1,2] This is followed by proximal involvement of the peroneus brevis, anterior tibialis, and digital extensors.[1] The strong peroneus longus and posterior tibialis muscles result in hindfoot varus and forefoot valgus/pronation.[2] Antagonists are the peroneus longus and the tibialis anterior. Therefore, in CMT, the anterior tibialis is relatively weak, thus the strong peroneus longus plantar flexes the first ray.[2] In addition, because the tibialis anterior is relatively weak, the extrinsic toe extensors dorsiflex in an attempt to compensate to cause hyperextension at the metatarsophalangeal joint.[2] Hyperextension at the metatarsophalangeal joint combined with flexion at the interphalangeal joint create a claw toe deformity.[1,2] Eventually the hindfoot goes into varus to restore a plantigrade foot also referred to as the tripod.[1,2] This causes the Achilles to become more medially located and act as a secondary hindfoot invertor.[1] As can be seen, the deformity has several mechanisms that create a positive feedback loop for cavovarus deformity, and the deformity worsens over time.

CLINICAL EVALUATION

Carovarus feet can present initially in children or adults, as flexible or fixed, and with or without overload in another part of the foot.[2] Clinical evaluation of patients with cavovarus foot deformity should include an extensive history with focus on birth history and family history.[1]

Physical examination should be performed in both the sitting and standing positions. In addition, the patient should be observed while walking. Specifically evaluate for callus location, stress fractures (most commonly of the fifth metatarsal from lateral column overload), claw toe deformity, Haglund's deformity or insertional Achilles tendinopathy (from Achilles tendon contracture), lateral ligament instability, peroneal pathology, and medial ankle or subtalar degenerative arthrosis.[1,2] Of these, the late findings are ankle instability, degenerative arthritis in the "triple-joint complex" (talonavicular, subtalar, and calcaneocuboid joints), in addition to varus talar tilt with resulting medial tibiotalar arthritis.[1,2] In addition, because hindfoot varus locks the transverse tarsal joints, the foot is not able to properly serve in shock absorption, which can result in medial tibial stress fractures as well as iliotibial band syndrome.[1]

An additional sign of hindfoot varus described by Beals and Manoli is the "peek-a-boo heel."[10] When viewing a normal foot from the front, the foot hides the heel, but in a cavus foot shape the medial heel is observable, hence the name peek-a-boo heel.

Charcot-Marie-Tooth patients may have calf atrophy, equinus during the swing phase, and a steppage gait.[1] The high-stepping drop-foot gait and knee hyperextension can result from secondary equinus at the ankle.[2] In CMT type 1A the most common presenting signs are areflexia and inability to perform the heel walk test.[1] Skre described late-onset sensory loss that is milder than motor loss in up to 25% of adults with CMT.[11]

Physical examination should also involve a complete neurologic examination including sensation, reflexes, and strength testing of muscles in the lower extremity.[2] If the patient presents with sensory loss, they are more prone to developing Charcot arthropathy in the foot or ankle.[1]

Another critical part of assessing hindfoot varus is the Coleman block test, which originated in 1997 (**Fig. 1**).[2,12] This test is used to determine if the hindfoot varus is driven by the forefoot as opposed to the intrinsics or tibialis posterior.[12] In addition, the Coleman block test determines if the deformity is flexible or fixed.[2] Another important method of evaluation is the Silfverskiold test, which should be used to determine if the inability to ankle dorsiflex originates from the heel cord or the gastroc-soleus complex.[2,13]

In the setting of congenital multiple arthrogryposis, the patient may present with a rigid, fixed equinovarus foot deformity. If the patient presents with a unilateral cavus foot, or if the foot deformity occurs with neurologic symptoms, evaluate for neuraxial abnormalities such as a spinal cord lesion, tethered cord, diastematomyelia, and myelomeningocele.[1,14] A high index of suspicion must exist because progression

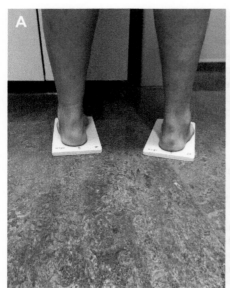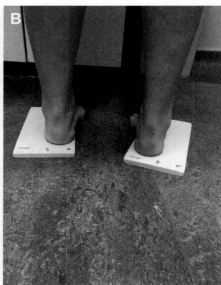

Fig. 1. Clinical photographs of the Coleman block test demonstrate (*A*) bilateral hindfoot varus standing alignment when the patient has her entire foot on the Coleman block. (*B*) When the patient's lateral foot is supported by the block, her hindfoot varus corrects, demonstrating that the hindfoot varus is driven by a plantarflexed first ray and that the deformity is flexible. (*Courtesy of* Dr Charles L. Saltzman, Salt Lake City, UT.)

of a cavus foot may be an indication for a tethered cord release.[14] In the setting of a unilateral cavovarus foot from peripheral nerve or spinal cord compression, the deformity is unlikely to progress significantly once the underlying problem is resolved.[3]

IMAGING

Radiographic evaluation begins with a weight-bearing anteroposterior and lateral (**Fig. 2**).[1,2] Calcaneal axial or hindfoot alignment views can help evaluate the position of the heel (**Fig. 3**).[15] Oblique views of the foot will assist in evaluation of the tarsometatarsal joints (**Fig. 4**).[2] On plain films, evaluate Meary's angle (talo-first metatarsal angle), which should be between 0° and 5°.[1] If Meary's angle has an apex dorsal, the foot is cavus. Other common signs of a cavovarus foot are a double talar dome sign (signifying that the talus is in external rotation), a see-through tarsal canal, and a wedge-shaped cuboid.[1] Osteophytes in the posterior subtalar joint can be a sign of early wear and tear of the subtalar joint.[2] With a diagnosis of CMT, consider ordering pelvic radiographs to evaluate for hip dysplasia and spine radiographs to evaluate for scoliosis, both associated conditions.[1] In addition to static images, fluoroscopic or ultrasound-guided anesthetic blocks may be useful to localize pain in patients.[2]

Advanced imaging should include a computed tomographic scan to evaluate arthritis, as well as for pre-operative planning.[1] More recently weight-bearing computed tomographic scans have been shown to be beneficial in evaluation of the anatomic relationship of bones during weight bearing.[16] Lastly, an MRI of the spine should be considered in the setting of unilateral cavus or spasticity.[1]

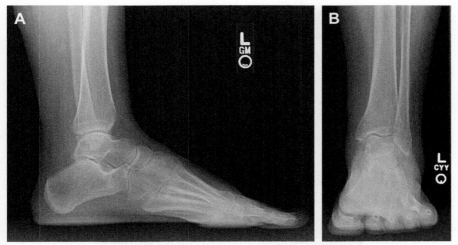

Fig. 2. Imaging evaluation of this left cavovarus foot deformity should include, at a minimum: (*A*) weight-bearing lateral and (*B*) anteroposterior radiographs of the ankle.

TREATMENT

Cavovarus foot deformity is actually a spectrum of deformities, therefore treatment should be individualized.[1] No 2 cavus feet are identical, thus it is difficult to propose a 1 size-fits-all treatment algorithm.[1] Treatment should focus on alleviating symptoms and restoring alignment of the hindfoot and forefoot to obtain a tripod foot.[1]

Non-Operative Management

Several different non-operative treatment modalities can be applied to cavovarus feet. These treatment modalities include physical therapy, lace-up ankle braces, orthotics with a cutout for the first metatarsal head and a lateral foot post (flexible deformities only), an ankle foot orthosis for foot drop and to prevent equinus contractures, night splints for tight heel cords and to prevent equinus, and shoe wear modification including wider toe boxes and extra depth, particularly for accommodation of claw toes.[1–3] Generally, it is difficult to fit high-arched feet into shoewear.[2] Rigid cavovarus feet probably will not do well with bracing or with hard orthotics, because neither change the deformity and instead are poorly tolerated and may predispose the patient to skin breakdown.[1,2]

Operative Management

Operative treatment includes soft tissue releases, tendon transfers, osteotomies, arthrodesis, and lateral ligament and peroneal tendon repairs or reconstructions.[1] Generally, joint sparing procedures should be attempted in skeletally immature patients or in adults with normal joints.[1,2] A general principle is that operative treatment should center around subtalar joint mobility.[1] Surgical timing depends on the etiology of the cavovarus foot deformity, the skeletal age of the patient, among others. Some surgeons are aggressive in proceeding with surgery, because the cavovarus clawfoot can be progressive in the setting of active muscle imbalances.[2] It is recommended to delay surgical intervention by 18 to 24 months in patients who have sustained a stroke because there is a possibility of functional recovery.[2] Generally, to correct muscular

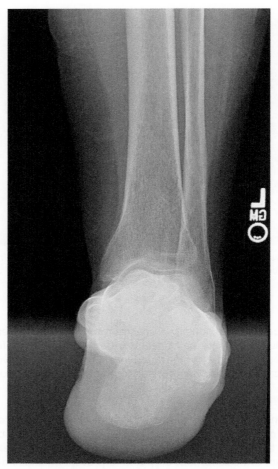

Fig. 3. Radiographic calcaneal axial or hindfoot alignment views of this left lower extremity can help evaluate the position of the heel.

imbalances, tendon transfers, osteotomies, and fusions are used. To correct rigid osseous deformity, use fusions and osteotomies.[2]

Soft tissue releases
Soft tissue releases typically include the plantar fascia, Achilles, and joint capsules of the subtalar and talonavicular joints.[1] Plantar fascial releases can be performed in cavovarus feet that are flexible or rigid, because in either case release permits dorsiflexion of the first ray.[1] When considering Achilles lengthening or gastrocnemius recession, caution must be exercised because weakness of ankle plantarflexors can cause permanent disability and is a risk associated with those procedures.[7]

Tendon transfers
There are many available tendon transfers. When deciding on which tendon transfer(s) to perform, in-phase transfers are preferable to out-of-phase transfers.[1] Two of the most common transfers performed are a full- or split-thickness tendon transfer of the posterior tibial tendon to the dorsum of the foot, as well as peroneus longus to

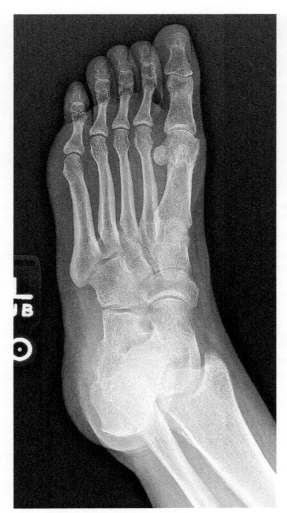

Fig. 4. The tarsometatarsal joints can be evaluated in his left foot through use of an oblique radiograph of the foot.

peroneus brevis. These are popular, as they reroute the 2 most deforming muscles in the cavovarus foot (tibialis posterior and peroneus longus).[2] There are several possible transfers in the forefoot, one of the most popular is the Jones transfer, which is transfer of the extensor hallicus longus to the dorsal aspect of the first metatarsal joint to assist the anterior tibialis tendon with dorsiflexion of the foot.

Osteotomy
Osteotomies generally include lateralizing the calcaneus and dorsiflexing the first ray.[2] A calcaneal osteotomy can pull the hindfoot out of varus. There are many different calcaneal osteotomies including: lateral calcaneal closing wedge osteotomy, lateralizing osteotomy, and L- or Z-type osteotomies.[1,17] In addition, there are many different forefoot and midfoot osteotomies and fusions to elevate the first ray to achieve a plantigrade foot.[1] The most common osteotomy is a dorsal closing wedge osteotomy of

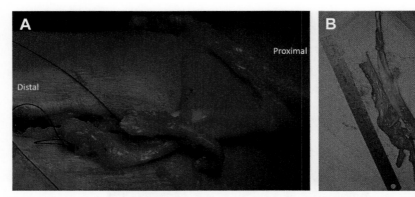

Fig. 5. (A) Intra-operative photographs from a left-sided peroneus brevis and longus resection in a cavovarus foot. (B) The peroneal tendons were excised and replaced with allograft.

the first metatarsal at the base, followed by a plantar opening wedge of the medial cuneiform.[1] In fact, combining these 2 osteotomies can correct up to 60° of cavus.[18] The authors of this article suggest reserving a tibial osteotomy for cases where the apex of the deformity is at the tibia.

Arthrodesis

Arthrodesis procedures are used as a salvage option or when there is late-stage destruction of joint spaces. Although a triple fusion has high rates of success, it also has high rates of adjacent joint disease.[1,2] Generally, arthrodesis is better for skeletally mature patients who have low physical demands and a rigid deformity.[1]

Other

If lateral ligament instability results from the cavovarus deformity, the modified Broström technique is a good solution if the remaining lateral ligament tissue is amenable.[1] If peroneal tendon pathology exists, the patient may need a peroneal debridement, repair, or replacement with allograft (**Fig. 5**).

SUMMARY

A cavovarus foot deformity results from muscle imbalances. There are several etiologies of a cavovarus foot, including congenital, neurologic, post-traumatic, and idiopathic. Charcot-Marie-Tooth disease is a common genetic cause of cavovarus foot. History, physical examination, and imaging help determine the appropriate treatment, which should be individualized to the patient. Non-operative management includes shoe wear modification, physical therapy, and bracing. Operative management consists of soft tissue releases, tendon transfers, osteotomies, arthrodesis, and lateral ligament or peroneal tendon repair or reconstruction.

REFERENCES

1. Georgiadis AG, Spiegel DA, Baldwin KD. The cavovarus foot in hereditary motor and sensory neuropathies. JBJS Rev 2015;3(12). https://doi.org/10.2106/JBJS. RVW.O.00024.
2. Younger AS, Hansen ST Jr. Adult cavovarus foot. J Am Acad Orthop Surg 2005; 13(5):302–15.

3. Beals TC, Nickisch F. Charcot-Marie-Tooth disease and the cavovarus foot. Foot Ankle Clin 2008;13(2):259–74, vi-vii.
4. Roa BB, Garcia CA, Suter U, et al. Charcot-Marie-Tooth disease type 1A. Association with a spontaneous point mutation in the PMP22 gene. N Engl J Med 1993; 329(2):96–101.
5. Charcot JM, Marie P. Sure one former particular d'atrophie musculaire progressive, souvent familiale débutant par les pieds et les jambes et atteignant plus tard les mains. Rev Med 1886;6:97–138.
6. Tooth HH. The peroneal type of progressive muscular atrophy. London: H.K. Lewis; 1886.
7. Beckmann NA, Wolf SI, Heitzmann D, et al. Cavovarus deformity in Charcot-Marie-Tooth disease: is there a hindfoot equinus deformity that needs treatment? J Foot Ankle Res 2015;8:65.
8. Wines AP, Chen D, Lynch B, et al. Foot deformities in children with hereditary motor and sensory neuropathy. J Pediatr Orthop 2005;25(2):241–4.
9. Tenuta J, Shelton YA, Miller F. Long-term follow-up of triple arthrodesis in patients with cerebral palsy. J Pediatr Orthop 1993;13(6):713–6.
10. Beals TC, Manoli A. The 'peek-a-boo' heel sign in the evaluation of hindfoot varus. Foot 1996;6(4):205–6.
11. Skre H. Genetic and clinical aspects of Charcot-Marie-Tooth's disease. Clin Genet 1974;6(2):98–118.
12. Coleman SS, Chesnut WJ. A simple test for hindfoot flexibility in the cavovarus foot. Clin Orthop Relat Res 1977;(123):60–2.
13. Silfverskiold N. Reduction of the uncrossed two-joints muscles of the leg to one-joint muscles in spastic conditions. Acta Chir Scand 1924;56:315–30.
14. Carpintero P, Entrenas R, Gonzalez I, et al. The relationship between pes cavus and idiopathic scoliosis. Spine (Phila Pa 1976) 1994;19(11):1260–3.
15. Saltzman CL, el-Khoury GY. The hindfoot alignment view. Foot Ankle Int 1995; 16(9):572–6.
16. Barg A, Bailey T, Richter M, et al. Weightbearing computed tomography of the foot and ankle: emerging technology topical review. Foot Ankle Int 2018;39(3): 376–86.
17. Malerba F, De Marchi F. Calcaneal osteotomies. Foot Ankle Clin 2005;10(3): 523–40, vii.
18. Mubarak SJ, Van Valin SE. Osteotomies of the foot for cavus deformities in children. J Pediatr Orthop 2009;29(3):294–9.

Updates in Pediatric Cavovarus Deformity

Kai Ziebarth, MD[a], Fabian Krause, MD[b],*

KEYWORDS

- Pediatric • Cavovarus deformity • Nonoperative • Operative • Treatment • Update

KEY POINTS

- The goal of the treatment of pediatric cavovarus deformities is a well-balanced foot with optimal plantar pressure distribution, no progression or recurrence of the deformity, and no or postponed concomitant ankle, midfoot, and hindfoot arthritis.
- The latest nonoperative measures are promising; however, if nonoperative treatment is unsatisfactory, surgical realignment has to be discussed with the patients and their parents.
- Recent publications demonstrate promising improvement in decision making and in operative techniques with good outcome.
- The current literature speaks in favor of an early and aggressive intervention to avoid progression of the deformity and concomitant consequences.

INTRODUCTION

The pediatric cavovarus deformity is often a 3-dimensional deformity caused by various underlying diseases. A thorough medical history and general examination of the patient regarding the primary disease is always necessary to understand the foot deformity. In the majority of cases, neurologic diseases are responsible for the deformity by causing muscular imbalance. In Charcot-Marie-Tooth (CMT) disease, the intrinsic foot muscles become weak and contracted while other foot muscles keep their physiologic strength. CMT accounts for about 66% of cavovarus cases,[1–4] but posttraumatic as well as residual clubfeet deformities have also been considered as possible causes for developing this deformity (**Box 1**[5]). For the treatment of cavovarus feet, it is important to know whether the underlying pathology will lead to a progressive deformity, because treatment strategies will be different and more demanding in progressive cases.

The authors have nothing to disclose.
[a] Department of Pediatric Surgery, Inselspital, University of Berne, Freiburgstrasse, 3010 Berne, Switzerland; [b] Department of Orthopaedic Surgery, Inselspital, University of Berne, Freiburgstrasse, 3010 Berne, Switzerland
* Corresponding author.
E-mail address: fabian.krause@insel.ch

> **Box 1**
> **Differential diagnosis for cavovarus foot deformity**
>
> Brain
>   Cerebral palsy
>   Friedrich's ataxia
>   Stroke
>   Tumor
>   Spinocerebellar degeneration
>
> Spinal cord
>   Tumor
>   Spinal dysraphism (tethered cord, myelomeningocele, diastematomyelia)
>   Poliomyelitis
>   Spinal muscular atrophy
>
> Peripheral nervous system
>   Hereditary sensorimotor neuropathy (eg, CMT)
>   Traumatic peripheral nerve lesions (sciatic nerve)
>
> Muscle and tendon
>   Leg compartment syndrome
>   Postsurgical clubfoot deformity
>   Peroneus longus tendon laceration
>   Duchenne muscular dystrophy
>
> Bone
>   Tarsal coalition
>   Malunion talar neck fracture
>
> Idiopathic
>
> *From* Lee MC, Sucato DJ. Pediatric issues with cavovarus foot deformities. Foot Ankle Clin 2008;13(2):199–219; with permission.

This article focuses on treatment options for cavovarus deformities in children that depend on the age of the patient and the localization of the anatomic pathology. It also summarizes treatment outcomes in the current literature to give an overview of which nonoperative measures or operative procedures might be most beneficial for young patients.

CLINICAL APPEARANCE

Ambulatory patients complain of muscle weakness, limited ankle dorsiflexion, and recurrent ankle sprains or progressing deformities of the foot and toes. In the majority of cases, there is a hindfoot varus malalignment accompanied by an elevated medial foot arch. Calluses along the lateral border of the foot and plantarly under the first and fifth metatarsal heads are common. Blisters or skin irritation over the dorsal aspect of the proximal interphalangeal joints of clawing toes are also often evident. In severe neurologic diseases (eg, cerebral palsy) with more or less nonambulatory patients, primarily flexible muscle contractures are responsible for the deformity that, over time, progress to rigid deformities impeding the positioning in braces. Thus, mobilization of the children for transfer from wheelchair to bed as well as for upright standing in a standing frame is not possible because the foot cannot be actively or passively placed in a neutral position.

In children younger than 10 years of age, the unloaded flexible foot occasionally seems to have a cavovarus deformity owing to an apparent elevated longitudinal arch, and the deformity disappears when in a weightbearing stance. These feet should be considered as a normal variant rather than a structural deformity. **Fig. 1** shows a 13-year-old boy with a fixed cavovarus deformity and a meningomyelocele. After several surgical procedures, a Lambrinudi operation was performed.

EXAMINATION

After a thorough general examination, the foot has to be inspected during gait and in the sitting and also weightbearing conditions, if possible. Any difference in size, abnormal callouses, or skin breakages are noted. The hindfoot alignment is observed from front and back. With regard to the underlying diagnosis, it is important to distinguish between a unilateral or bilateral deformity (see **Box 1**).

The function and aspect of each part of the foot is examined and range of motion, particularly of the ankle, subtalar, and Chopart's joints, is documented. The function and position of the forefoot midfoot and hindfoot in relation to each other is also looked at. The ankle is examined for ligamentous instability by an anterior drawer test and lateral talar tilt. The amplitude and strength of the tendons and respective muscles must be analyzed. Especially in neurologic disorders, a muscular imbalance is common. The Coleman block[6–8] test is routinely performed in the examination for cavovarus feet.

Static and dynamic pedobarographic analysis and documentation of deformity progression allow for a reliable evaluation and postoperative comparison if surgery is considered[9] (**Fig. 1**). It often helps to identify the zones of overloading more precisely. Referral to a gait laboratory might be required in complex cases where the general pathology of the lower extremity has to be evaluated. Dreher and colleagues[10] stated that a major limitation of conventional gait analysis models when evaluating foot deformities is their representation of the foot as a single rigid lever. They prefer to use a kinematic foot model.[11]

Standard anteroposterior and lateral weightbearing radiographs of the foot and a Mortise view of the ankle are sufficient in the majority of cases. Anteroposterior and lateral (Meary's) talo–first metatarsal angle as well as the calcaneal pitch angle are appropriate radiographic parameters to evaluate the deformity's location, extent, and progression. Also, an assessment of bone quality and deformity-related changes of bone morphology during growth is important when surgery is needed.

Only if the foot deformity or the extent of cartilage damage and arthritis remain unclear from plain radiographs should MRI or a computed tomography scan of the foot and ankle come into play. MRI and a computed tomography scan will help to decide

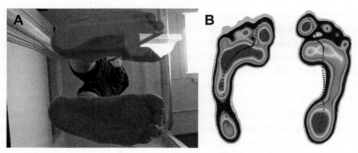

Fig. 1. (*A, B*) Right clubfoot of a 13-year-old boy standing on a podoscope. The left foot is healthy (*A*). Pedobarographic load analysis (Zebris Medical GmbH, Isny, Germany) of the same patient (*B*).

whether a joint preserving surgery is still possible or joint sacrificing midfoot and hind-foot arthrodesis has to be made. However, if a tethered cord or other spinal pathologies are expected, an MRI of the spine is always required.

TREATMENT

If the forefoot is flexible, orthotics and soft tissue procedures should be considered first for ambulatory patients. Plantar release and various tendon transfers can be used in more flexible feet. However, the recent literature for the operative treatment of cavovarus feet in children favors an early and aggressive intervention to avoid progression of the deformity. The importance to correct the muscle imbalance is acknowledged by most authors but inconsistently interpreted. Wicart and Seringe[1] do not include any tendon transfer in their bony and soft-tissue realignment; Mosca[12] considers the peroneus longus transfer obligatorily but avoids the tibialis posterior transfer; and Kumar and colleagues[13] prefer the tibialis posterior transfer without the peroneus longus transfer.

In nonambulatory patients, the goal of treatment is a plantigrade foot to allow bed to wheelchair transfer or short mobilization with braces/orthotics in an upright position or in a standing frame. The level of activity with the ambulatory status, general condition, and bone or soft tissue quality are important factors when indicating and planning surgery.

Nonoperative Treatment

The literature regarding the nonoperative treatment of cavovarus deformity in children is scarce. Depending on the severity of the cavovarus deformity, a stretching of the contracted plantar structures by physiotherapy and load-distributing, unloading orthotics in combination with shoe modifications may be helpful. Historically, the effectiveness of nonoperative treatment has been controversial.[14,15] Recent studies demonstrate that nonoperative treatment is effective, especially for very young children.[16,17] Even though the effectiveness of stretching in patients with cerebral palsy is limited,[18] current treatment strategies should include physiotherapy as adjunct procedures in any underlying neurologic diseases. In a recent randomized, controlled study by Maas and colleagues,[19] a knee–ankle–foot orthosis used to prevent progressive loss of motion was not well-tolerated and did not prevent a progressive decrease in ankle motion over time in children with cerebral palsy.

d'Astorg and colleagues,[16] however, reported 65% good and very good results at a mean follow-up of 4.5 for patients who used an untwisting walking casts for 6 weeks postoperatively followed by a nocturnal untwisting splint in neurologic cavovarus deformities in children. Surgery was either avoided or postponed by a mean 4.5 years, allowing surgical treatment in a single step before the end of growth.

Because, in CMT disease, a muscle imbalance causes the cavovarus deformity, the injection of botulinum toxin into the stronger muscle seems to be a reasonable treatment approach. In 2010, Burns and colleagues[20] studied the application of 7 IU/kg botulinum toxin injection in the tibialis posterior and peroneus longus muscle every 6 months to prevent the cavovarus deformity progression in 10 children with CMT in a noncontrolled, randomized trial. However, 2 years after the index injection, there was no significant decrease in the deformity progression in the treated leg as opposed to the untreated leg. In a case report, however, Tiffreau and colleagues[21] presented a 12-year-old girl suffering from CMT in whom progressive pes cavovarus was relieved by 50 IU botulinum toxin injection into the posterior tibialis muscle over a period of 6 months. In both studies, the toxin injections did not seem to have adverse events.

Nonoperative treatment fails with progression of the anatomic alterations of the foot and increasing pain or limited daily activity of the patient.

Operative Treatment

Release of the plantar fascia

If surgery for the cavovarus deformity is required in the child, plantar fascia release in combination with osteotomies is the common procedure nowadays. In younger children with a flexible hindfoot, a plantar release as a single operation may flatten the longitudinal arch in mild deformities. Plantar release can be performed percutaneously or open. Especially in moderate or severe cases, an open radical plantar release is recommended.[9] Postoperative treatment includes serial casting to retain the foot position that was achieved intraoperatively and to stretch the plantar structures to prevent recurrence. Plantar release might be considered in almost all surgical variations for the treatment of cavovarus deformities, because the plantar fascia is contracted in almost all cases of the deformity. Although some surgeons introduce plantar fascia release as a single treatment in mild to moderate deformities,[22] Kwon and colleagues[6] recently presented a better foot pressure distribution if plantar fascia release is combined with a first metatarsal osteotomy. In a pilot study, Sanpera and associates[23] combined a plantar fascia release with a dorsal hemiepiphysiodesis of the first metatarsal with a sufficient correction after a median of 28 months. Some authors recommend the introduction of an external ring fixation to distract the soft tissue and to realign the foot.[24–26] If the deformity is only partially corrected by an external fixator, osteotomies of the midfoot are commonly added.

Tendon transfer

Because most patients with a cavovarus deformity have an underlying neurologic disease, the indication for tendon transfers to relieve muscular imbalance is reasonable. Because the muscle strength is not physiologic and might be progressive, the effect of the tendon transfer is barely predictable. Thus, tendon transfers should be considered carefully after a thorough examination of the muscle strength; a referral to a pediatric neurologist is recommended before surgery. With every tendon transfer, a loss of at least 1 grade of strength has to be considered. With regard to the gait cycle, in-phase transfers are generally more efficient than out-of-phase transfers, especially in the case of younger child whose brain demonstrates an enormous capacity to adapt.

Transfer of the peroneus longus to brevis muscle is commonly combined with additional bony surgery. It removes the plantar flexion force of the peroneus longus muscle from the proximal first metatarsal bone, while reinforcing the eversion of the peroneus brevis muscle. Also, the function of the weak anterior tibialis muscle may be indirectly improved.

In patients with muscular dystrophies or peripheral neuropathies, the anterior tibialis muscle cannot dorsiflex the ankle satisfactorily. Hence, the strong tibialis posterior muscle induces hindfoot varus deformity. In this situation, a transfer of the posterior tibialis tendon to the anterior tibialis tendon may help the patient to better dorsiflex the foot. It also helps in correcting the hindfoot varus indirectly. Dreher and co-workers[10] found the tibialis posterior transfer to be effective in patients with cavovarus deformity owing to CMT disease. In their study, the tibialis posterior muscle was divided and transferred to the tibialis anterior and the peroneus brevis muscle, respectively. They showed an improvement of the ankle dorsiflexion during swing phase in the 3-dimensional gait analysis; plantarflexion and push off were weakened. It has to be noted that a tendon transfer can infrequently create a secondary deformity if the muscle imbalance turns in the opposite direction (eg, by overstrengthening of dorsiflexion and valgization forces in cerebral palsy), leading to calcaneovalgus deformity.

If surgery is required in children with cerebral palsy, some authors have recommend that, if the deformity is present during the stance phase, about one-half of the overactive tibialis posterior should be transferred to the peroneus brevis. One-half of the tibialis anterior transfer is indicated in the case of dynamic supination of the foot during the swing phase.[27] A transfer of the entire tibialis posterior is not suggested for young, diplegic patients with poor ambulation because of the risk of poor outcomes owing to an overcorrection into a permanent planovalgus deformity.

The indication for a Jones transfer is given only in flexible cavovarus deformity without a rigid varus of the hindfoot and consists of a transfer of the extensor hallucis longus and brevis muscle to the metatarsal head. This operation was modified by several authors and combined with interphalangeal arthrodesis and dorsiflexion proximal first metatarsal osteotomy. Breusch and colleagues[28] reported satisfying results in 86% of 51 patients (81 feet) at a mean follow-up of 42 months. The indication was neurologic cavovarus deformity in the majority of cases.

Erickson and colleagues[29] treated flexible cavovarus feet (19 patients with CMT; 30 feet; average age of 12 years) with soft tissue procedures only, including Steindler stripping, plantar fascia release, posterior tibialis tendon transfer, Jones tendon transfer, and Achilles lengthening. At an average follow-up of 2.6 years, they recorded mainly significant improvements in radiographic and pedobarographic measures. However, pressure distributions did not fully normalize. The authors concluded that ongoing high peak pressures under the first metatarsal head could indicate the need for a more aggressive correction of the first metatarsal plantarflexion. Interestingly, 1 foot was overcorrected into a planovalgus deformity, but the patient remained asymptomatic.

Isolated first ray dorsiflexion osteotomies

Although plantar fascia release is generally combined with first metatarsal dorsiflexion osteotomies,[5] Singh and Briggs[30] (2012) reported good results in first metatarsal osteotomies even without plantar release. The proximal first metatarsal osteotomy is traditionally performed in a dorsal closing wedge fashion. In younger children, the proximal physis of the first metatarsal must be protected. In severe deformities, the osteotomy of the remaining metatarsals might be necessary. A more proximal dorsiflexion osteotomy of the medial cuneiform (reversed Cotton osteotomy) allows a more powerful correction in theory but is restricted by the Lisfranc's ligament. Also, the fixation of the medial cuneiform osteotomy often is more challenging than the fixation of the proximal first metatarsal.

The long-term results of 25 adolescents with CMT and cavovarus deformity that had dorsiflexion osteotomy of the first metatarsal, transfer of the peroneus longus to the peroneus brevis, plantar fascia release, transfer of the extensor hallucis longus to the neck of the first metatarsal, and, in selected cases, transfer of the tibialis anterior tendon to the lateral cuneiform were encouraging at average follow-up of 26 years. Although the Short Form-36 physical component score was lower than age-matched norms and moderate to severe arthritis was observed in 11 feet, no patient required a triple fusion.[31]

Combined midfoot osteotomies (joint sparing)

Severe and rigid cavovarus deformities are the main indication for midfoot osteotomies. They should also be combined with a plantar fascia release to allow sufficient correction.[5] The age of the patient for bony procedures should be 8 years or older to prevent an excessive shortening of the foot after surgery by affecting the growth of the respective bones of the midfoot. In a recent study, Elgeidi and Abulsaad[32] executed a combined double tarsal wedge and transcuneiform osteotomy in children between 4 and 9 years of age for residual cavovarus after severe clubfoot deformity. They did not report any growth disturbances of the feet at 5 years postoperatively. Thus, if a patient is suffering from the deformity and quality of life is strongly reduced, the cut-off age can be lowered in exceptional cases. The indication for a bony procedure in a very young child must be individually discussed with the parents regarding complications like growth disturbance of the foot.

Several operative techniques for midfoot osteotomies have been published. Depending on the individual cavovarus pattern, the decision to perform an opening or closing wedge osteotomy is made. Because the apex of the midfoot deformity is in the naviculocuneiform joint or in the cuneiforms itself, dorsiflexion of the first ray is currently achieved by a combination of the abovementioned first metatarsal dorsiflexion osteotomy with a plantar opening wedge osteotomy of the first cuneiform.

Mubarak and Van Valin[33] recommended a joint-sparing stepwise procedure for the correction of severe cavovarus deformity by combining metatarsal, cuneiform, and calcaneal osteotomies depending on the deformity pattern. The first step usually was a 20° to 30° plantar opening wedge osteotomy of the medial cuneiform in combination with a 20° to 30° dorsal closing wedge osteotomy of the first metatarsal using the metatarsal wedge to fill the cuneiform gap. Almost all patients underwent a 5- to 10-mm closing wedge osteotomy of the cuboid to correct the forefoot adductus and to support forefoot dorsiflexion. In about 25% of cases, a dorsal closing wedge metatarsal osteotomy was added if plantar prominence of the second and third metatarsal heads was palpable. A closing wedge calcaneal osteotomy with lateralization of the calcaneal tuberosity was used for a fixed hindfoot varus. The average age of patients in their study was 11 years and the mean follow-up was 46 months. No severe complication occurred, and the radiographic alignment as well as the clinical appearance improved.

Also, Mosca[12] advocated a plantar opening wedge cuneiform osteotomy instead of first metatarsal osteotomy, because the cuneiform is closer to the apex of the deformity. An additional advantage of the plantar-based open wedge deformity is to better correct the forefoot adduction by spreading the medial osteotomy gap of the cuneiform bone more medially than laterally because of the intermetatarsal ligaments. Hence, in cases with excessive forefoot adduction, a plantar-based osteotomy is indicated, whereas in cases with only little forefoot adduction a dorsal closed wedge osteotomy maybe sufficient as well. Wicart and Seringe[34] published promising results of a similar operation technique in 26 neurogenic cavovarus feet at a mean follow up of 6.9 years. The authors performed opening wedge (cuneiform I–III) midfoot osteotomies combined with plantar fascia release and lateral sliding calcaneal osteotomy.

Calcaneal osteotomies

In cavovarus deformities with a rigid hindfoot as assessed by the Coleman bloc test, a calcaneal osteotomy is indicated to reduce or neutralize the varus alignment of the hindfoot. Different techniques are available but the lateral sliding and closing wedge (Dwyer) osteotomy[35] or the calcaneal sliding osteotomy seem to be preferred treatment of many surgeons. Results of this osteotomy are promising, as mentioned, in combination with midfoot osteotomies.[33,34,36] One of the disadvantages of the Dwyer osteotomy is the relative lengthening of the Achilles tendon, which may weaken the push off force while walking if a concomitant tibialis posterior transfer was performed.

A medial open wedge calcaneal osteotomy should not be considered owing to the problem of wound healing, even in children.

Midfoot osteotomies (joint sacrificing)/midfoot arthrodesis

In older children with rigid deformities where the aforementioned options are no longer applicable, the deformity must be corrected through the joints or by arthrodesis. Because CMT is a progressive disease, the recurrence of the cavovarus deformity requiring triple arthrodeses ranges between 30% and 80% despite diverse operative approaches with bony and soft tissue procedures.[1] In the past, many patients with cavovarus deformity and CMT were treated with triple arthrodesis as a definitive procedure to generate a well-aligned, functional foot. However, long-term follow-up studies reported a high incidence of arthritis of the adjacent joints after this procedure.[37]

Different techniques of midfoot osteotomies are known to correct rigid cavovarus deformities (eg, the Japas V-osteotomy) as well as the dorsal closing midfoot osteotomy through the Chopart joint[38,39] or the Lambrinudi technique.[24] Mubarak and Dimeglio[40] described a salvage procedure for failed previous realignment procedures. The authors excised the navicular bone and performed a dorsal closing wedge midfoot osteotomy through the cuboid. Results of this salvage procedure were good at the 5-year follow-up.

If a sufficient correction of the cavovarus cannot be achieved despite multiple previous surgeries or the disease itself damaged the cartilage of the respective joints, triple arthrodesis must be considered. The goal of an arthrodesis is to correct the foot into a neutral plantar position (**Fig. 2**). Again, the long-term results of triple arthrodesis

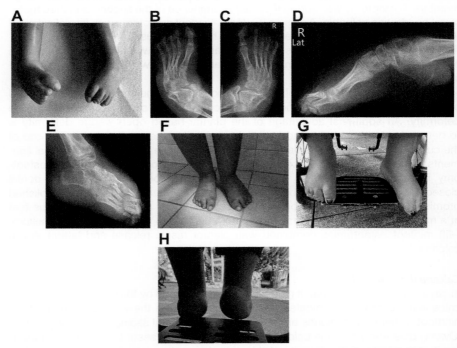

Fig. 2. A 13-year-old girl with MMC (meningomyelocele). Outcome after bilateral derotation osteotomy tibia. Owing to the deformity of the feet, transfer bed wheelchair and mobilizing in standing frame was difficult. (*A*) Clinical status preoperatively (*B–E*). Preoperative radiographs. (*F–H*) Postoperative clinical picture after triple arthrodesis.

have shown further deterioration by adjacent joint arthritis in the long term.[37] The surgeon should be aware of numerous complications (eg, nonunion or loss of alignment, particularly in patients with neurologic diseases).

Zhou and colleagues[41] published good outcomes for 17 adolescents and young adults (12–36 years of age) after the Cole-type midfoot osteotomy; this osteotomy consists of a naviculocuneiform wedge-shaped osteotomy with fusion and a wedge-shaped osteotomy of the cuboid in combination with a percutaneous plantar fascia release for a rigid cavovarus deformity. In some patients, the posterior tibial tendon was transferred selectively through the interosseous membrane to the dorsum of the foot using a suture anchor. In the case of an equinus contracture, a Z-plasty of the Achilles tendon was performed. Claw toes were aligned in extension with K-wires usually after tenotomy of the respective flexor tendons. An arthrodesis of the distal phalangeal joint is rarely indicated (only in fixed deformities).

GENERAL REMARKS
Nonambulatory Patients

Because these patients are constantly nonweightbearing (eg, wheelchair or bedridden) the bone quality is poor. When considering osteotomies or arthrodesis the surgeon needs to be aware of this fact. The alignment with opening wedge osteotomies are more difficult to retain than closing wedge osteotomies because the weak bone will likely at least partially collapse, even with cortical bone grafting. If an arthrodesis is performed, the fixation of the respective bones by wires, screws, or plates is critical, even with new and modern implants. Therefore, postoperative longtime casting with concomitant bracing is necessary to achieve bone healing with appropriate stability. As mentioned, there are several techniques for midfoot osteotomies reported in literature. However, in some cases the surgeon has to judge intraoperatively about the precise direction of the osteotomy line because the midfoot bones are joined together like a single bone block hampering the intraoperative identification even with the image intensifier. Thus, osteotomies in nonambulatory patients sometimes have to be modified owing to the intraoperative anatomic situation.

Ambulatory Patients

Residual clubfoot deformities
The first choice for residual clubfoot deformity, even in the case of older children, is another series of casting[42] before considering surgery. For a persistent cavovarus deformity in children older than 3 years of age, indications for tendon transfer and/or osteotomies are published.[32] It is very important to differentiate a dynamic supination from a cavovarus deformity. In a dynamic supination case, the tibialis anterior transfer is a well-known and successful operation. The transfer can be performed as soon the ossified nucleus of the lateral cuneiform is visible at the age of 3 to 4 years. In syndrome clubfeet, a posteromedial release sometimes with lateral release is inevitable. However, in idiopathic clubfeet, a residual cavovarus deformity might be treated by plantar fascia release and selective tendon transfer or first metatarsal osteotomy according to patients with CMT.

Charcot-Marie-Tooth patients
Meticulous examination and localization of the apex of the deformity helps in the decision making for surgery. A modified Jones or plantar open wedge osteotomies of the first cuneiform are commonly used with concomitant tendon transfer, as discussed elsewhere in this article. In the case of fixed hindfoot varus deformity, the closed wedge Dwyer osteotomy is recommended (**Fig. 3**). Because the tibial nerve can be

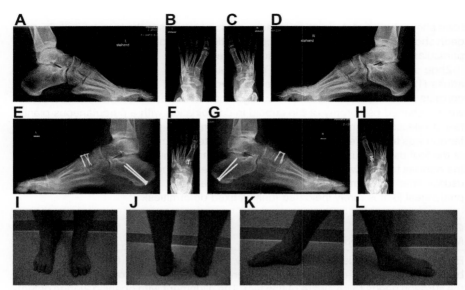

Fig. 3. A 15-year-old boy with CMT type 1A disease. He experienced recurrent ankle sprains and pressure marks on the skin, as well as pain over the dorsum of the feet. (*A–H*) Preoperative and postoperative radiographs after a bilateral closed wedge cuneiform 3 osteotomy and valgus sliding calcaneal osteotomy, transfer of two-thirds of the M tibialis posterior to the navicular bone, tenodesis of the M peroneus longus to brevis, and Z-lengthening of the Achilles tendon. (*I–L*) Clinical status postoperatively.

entrapped underneath the flexor retinaculum after the calcaneal osteotomy, an open tibial release to prevent neurologic complications has to be considered in the same settings.

Tethered cord
In the case of tethered cord syndrome, the myelon has to be untethered before corrective surgery for cavovarus deformity is planned. It is reasonable to wait a few months to observe the development of the deformity of the foot after the detethering procedure. Sometimes bracing and stretching will reduce the deformity and surgery can be postponed or even canceled. If surgical correction is foreseen, a combined procedure of tendon transfer and a joint-sparing osteotomy is introduced.

Cerebral palsy
Patients with cerebral palsy or severe muscular imbalance owing to other neurologic problems are difficult to treat with joint-sparing procedures depending on the severity of the disease. In general, nonoperative treatment (eg, bracing) provides delay for surgical treatment. Tendon transfers may contribute to realignment by bony procedures at an early stage, but they may have an adverse effect by changing the imbalance in the opposite direction, leading to an overcorrection of the deformity. Most feet may end up requiring an arthrodesis, mainly triple arthrodesis. For stretching of the soft tissue before osteotomies or even partial or complete reduction of the deformity itself, an external fixation might be helpful in some cases.

SUMMARY

The goal of the treatment of pediatric cavovarus deformities is to neutralize plantar pressure distribution, reduce the hindfoot varus deformity, and avoid or postpone hindfoot arthritis. Recent nonoperative measures (eg, botulinum toxin injections) hold promise to achieve this goal. However, if nonoperative treatment is not an option, surgical realignment has to be discussed with the patients and their parents. Several improvements in indications and techniques have been published recently. However, to avoid disappointment in patients owing to a recurrence of the deformity and symptoms or several failures of operative procedures, selection of the appropriate and preferably single operative procedure at the appropriate time point of the child's development remains the most crucial factor for a successful treatment.

Reviewing the literature there are no evidence-based guidelines available for the successful treatment of cavovarus deformities in children. The individual pattern of cavovarus deformity and the underlying disease in ambulatory or nonambulatory patient influence the respective treatment and have to be considered if a surgical correction is planned.

REFERENCES

1. Wicart P. Cavus foot, from neonates to adolescents. Orthop Traumatol Surg Res 2012;98(7):813–28.
2. Ghanem I, Zeller R, Seringe R. The foot in hereditary motor and sensory neuropathies in children. Rev Chir Orthop Reparatrice Appar Mot 1996;82(2):152–60 [in French].
3. Laura M, Singh D, Ramdharry G, et al. Prevalence and orthopedic management of foot and ankle deformities in Charcot-Marie-Tooth disease. Muscle Nerve 2018; 57(2):255–9.
4. Olney B. Treatment of the cavus foot. Deformity in the pediatric patient with Charcot-Marie-Tooth. Foot Ankle Clin 2000;5(2):305–15.
5. Lee MC, Sucato DJ. Pediatric issues with cavovarus foot deformities. Foot Ankle Clin 2008;13(2):199–219, v.
6. Kwon YU, Kim HW, Hwang JH, et al. Changes in dynamic pedobarography after extensive plantarmedial release for paralytic pes cavovarus. Yonsei Med J 2014; 55(3):766–72.
7. Coleman SS, Chesnut WJ. A simple test for hindfoot flexibility in the cavovarus foot. Clin Orthop Relat Res 1977;(123):60–2.
8. Myers SR. A simple test for hindfoot flexibility in the cavovarus foot. Clin Orthop Relat Res 1990;(258):310.
9. Hamel J. Corrective procedures and indications for cavovarus foot deformities in children and adolescents. Oper Orthop Traumatol 2017;29(6):473–82 [in German].
10. Dreher T, Wolf SI, Heitzmann D, et al. Tibialis posterior tendon transfer corrects the foot drop component of cavovarus foot deformity in Charcot-Marie-Tooth disease. J Bone Joint Surg Am 2014;96(6):456–62.
11. Stebbins J, Harrington M, Thompson N, et al. Repeatability of a model for measuring multi-segment foot kinematics in children. Gait Posture 2006;23(4): 401–10.
12. Mosca VS. The cavus foot. J Pediatr Orthop 2001;21(4):423–4.
13. Myung K. Cavus deformity. In: The child's foot and ankle. 2nd edition. Philadelphia: Lippincott; 2009. p. 174–87.
14. McCluskey WP, Lovell WW, Cummings RJ. The cavovarus foot deformity. Etiology and management. Clin Orthop Relat Res 1989;(247):27–37.

15. Paulos L, Coleman SS, Samuelson KM. Pes cavovarus. Review of a surgical approach using selective soft-tissue procedures. J Bone Joint Surg Am 1980; 62(6):942–53.
16. d'Astorg H, Rampal V, Seringe R, et al. Is non-operative management of childhood neurologic cavovarus foot effective? Orthop Traumatol Surg Res 2016; 102(8):1087–91.
17. Watanabe K. Treatment for patients with Charcot-Marie-Tooth disease: orthopaedic aspects. Brain Nerve 2016;68(1):51–7 [in Japanese].
18. Pin T, Dyke P, Chan M. The effectiveness of passive stretching in children with cerebral palsy. Dev Med Child Neurol 2006;48(10):855–62.
19. Maas J, Dallmeijer A, Huijing P, et al. A randomized controlled trial studying efficacy and tolerance of a knee-ankle-foot orthosis used to prevent equinus in children with spastic cerebral palsy. Clin Rehabil 2014;28(10):1025–38.
20. Burns J, Scheinberg A, Ryan MM, et al. Randomized trial of botulinum toxin to prevent pes cavus progression in pediatric Charcot-Marie-Tooth disease type 1A. Muscle Nerve 2010;42(2):262–7.
21. Tiffreau V, Allart E, Dangleterre C, et al. Botulinum toxin treatment of pes cavovarus in a child suffering from autosomal recessive axonal Charcot-Marie-Tooth neuropathy (AR-CMT2). Eur J Phys Rehabil Med 2015;51(3):345–9.
22. Sherman FC, Westin GW. Plantar release in the correction of deformities of the foot in childhood. J Bone Joint Surg Am 1981;63(9):1382–9.
23. Sanpera I Jr, Frontera-Juan G, Sanpera-Iglesias J, et al. Innovative treatment for pes cavovarus: a pilot study of 13 children. Acta Orthop 2018;89(6):668–73.
24. Hall JE, Calvert PT. Lambrinudi triple arthrodesis: a review with particular reference to the technique of operation. J Pediatr Orthop 1987;7(1):19–24.
25. Kucukkaya M, Kabukcuoglu Y, Kuzgun U. Management of the neuromuscular foot deformities with the Ilizarov method. Foot Ankle Int 2002;23(2):135–41.
26. Hosny GA. Correction of foot deformities by the Ilizarov method without corrective osteotomies or soft tissue release. J Pediatr Orthop B 2002;11(2):121–8.
27. Scott AC, Scarborough N. The use of dynamic EMG in predicting the outcome of split posterior tibial tendon transfers in spastic hemiplegia. J Pediatr Orthop 2006;26(6):777–80.
28. Breusch SJ, Wenz W, Doderlein L. Function after correction of a clawed great toe by a modified Robert Jones transfer. J Bone Joint Surg Br 2000;82(2):250–4.
29. Erickson S, Hosseinzadeh P, Iwinski HJ, et al. Dynamic pedobarography and radiographic evaluation of surgically treated cavovarus foot deformity in children with Charcot-Marie-Tooth disease. J Pediatr Orthop 2015;24(4):336–40.
30. Singh AK, Briggs PJ. Metatarsal extension osteotomy without plantar aponeurosis release in cavus feet. The effect on claw toe deformity a radiographic assessment. Foot Ankle Surg 2012;18(3):210–2.
31. Ward CM, Dolan LA, Bennett DL, et al. Long-term results of reconstruction for treatment of a flexible cavovarus foot in Charcot-Marie-Tooth disease. J Bone Joint Surg Am 2008;90(12):2631–42.
32. Elgeidi A, Abulsaad M. Combined double tarsal wedge osteotomy and transcuneiform osteotomy for correction of resistant clubfoot deformity (the "bean-shaped" foot). J Child Orthop 2014;8(5):399–404.
33. Mubarak SJ, Van Valin SE. Osteotomies of the foot for cavus deformities in children. J Pediatr Orthop 2009;29(3):294–9.
34. Wicart P, Seringe R. Plantar opening-wedge osteotomy of cuneiform bones combined with selective plantar release and Dwyer osteotomy for pes cavovarus in children. J Pediatr Orthop 2006;26(1):100–8.

35. Dwyer FC. Osteotomy of the calcaneum for pes cavus. J Bone Joint Surg Br 1959;41-B(1):80–6.
36. Silver CM, Simon SD, Litchman HM. Long term follow-up observations on calcaneal osteotomy. Clin Orthop Relat Res 1974;(99):181–7.
37. Saltzman CL, Fehrle MJ, Cooper RR, et al. Triple arthrodesis: twenty-five and forty-four-year average follow-up of the same patients. J Bone Joint Surg Am 1999;81(10):1391–402.
38. Cole WH. The classic. The treatment of claw-foot. By Wallace H. Cole. 1940. Clin Orthop Relat Res 1983;(181):3–6.
39. Japas LM. Surgical treatment of pes cavus by tarsal V-osteotomy. Preliminary report. J Bone Joint Surg Am 1968;50(5):927–44.
40. Mubarak SJ, Dimeglio A. Navicular excision and cuboid closing wedge for severe cavovarus foot deformities: a salvage procedure. J Pediatr Orthop 2011;31(5):551–6.
41. Zhou Y, Zhou B, Liu J, et al. A prospective study of midfoot osteotomy combined with adjacent joint sparing internal fixation in treatment of rigid pes cavus deformity. J Orthop Surg Res 2014;9:44.
42. Dragoni M, Farsetti P, Vena G, et al. Ponseti treatment of rigid residual deformity in congenital clubfoot after walking age. J Bone Joint Surg Am 2016;98(20):1706–12.

Inframalleolar Varus Deformity
Role of Calcaneal Osteotomies

Federico Giuseppe Usuelli, MD*, Luigi Manzi, MD

KEYWORDS

- Joint-preserving surgery • Cavo varus foot classification • Calcaneal osteotomy
- Supramalleolar osteotomies • Hindfoot alignment • Pes cavus • Cavovarus foot

KEY POINTS

- Clinical examination is key to identifying any functional loss.
- Weight-bearing radiographs are used for procedure selection and quantifying the required correction.
- Although several calcaneal osteotomies have been previously proposed to correct varus heel deformities, the modified sliding-Z-shaped osteotomy appears to be a very powerful tool for correction.
- Cavo varus foot is a challenging pathology and a rigorous algorithm of treatment is necessary.
- In case of inframalleolar ankle deformities, the calcaneal osteotomy represents a tool that may be used in combination with different procedures to achieve a well-aligned foot and ankle complex.

INTRODUCTION

The cavus foot is a very complex deformity.

It is reported to affect approximately 20% to 25% of the population.[1]

The cavus shape induces deep biomechanical changings in the foot and ankle complex. The eventual deformities are the result of an imbalance between the intrinsic and extrinsic muscles. This is the mechanism in charge of osteoarticular malalignment and consequent gross deformities.

Neurologic diseases[2] are more frequently responsible for these deformities (Charcot-Marie-Tooth disease, cerebral palsy, poliomyelitis); however, posttraumatic, residual clubfoot, and idiopathic[3] are other common reasons for a cavo varus foot.

Disclosures: Dr F.G. Usuelli: consultant for Zimmer-Biomet, Geistlich. Dr L. Manzi has no disclosures.
C.A.S.C.O. Foot and Ankle Unit, IRCCS Galeazzi, Via Riccardo Galeazzi, 20161 Milan, Italy
* Corresponding author.
E-mail address: fusuelli@gmail.com

Foot Ankle Clin N Am 24 (2019) 219–237
https://doi.org/10.1016/j.fcl.2019.02.011

Cavo varus deformity can be classified according to flexibility and severity of the malalignment, ranging from a subtle and flexible cavo varus foot, as described by Manoli and Graham,[4] to a severe cavo varus posture accompanied by fixed bony malalignment.

More recently, some investigators proposed to study the whole complex of the foot and ankle when approaching the cavus foot. They stressed the principle that a limited prospective, focused solely on the hindfoot, limits understanding of the pathology.[5,6]

Furthermore, subtalar and talonavicular joints have been shown to provide greater compensation for proximal deformities (ankle, knee, and total limb).[7]

These findings may explain the increasing interest toward hindfoot and inframalleolar deformity correlation, which introduces new indications for calcaneal osteotomies.

A comprehensive classification is still needed and may be useful for defining an algorithm of treatment.

Such an algorithm has already been successfully implemented for flat foot deformities and posterior tibial tendon dysfunctions with a positive impact on clinical practice by Myerson and Bluman and other authors.[8–10]

Treatment options for the cavus foot include soft tissue procedures (ligament reconstruction and tendon transfers) and bone corrections (osteotomies and fusions).

This article reviews the several surgical options for calcaneal osteotomies and proposes a comprehensive algorithm of treatment, considering the whole foot and ankle complex.

BIOMECHANICS OF THE FOOT AND ANKLE COMPLEX

Ankle and hindfoot malalignment is the most important feature in the cavo varus foot. It is driven by a muscle imbalance between agonist and antagonist. The final result is the overpowering of one function by the other, inducing dysfunction and eventually deformity.

Biomechanically, "cavus" is defined as a varus hindfoot, high-pitched midfoot, plantar-flexed, and adducted forefoot. This condition depends on posterior tibial tendon strength and contraction, resulting in varus hindfoot alignment and midfoot and forefoot adduction, whereas the peroneus brevis may be weak or even absent.[11]

Varus malalignment at the heel results in a medial pulling vector of the Achilles tendon, increasing the inversion moment. Moreover, a weak tibialis anterior muscle results in an overpowered peroneus longus muscle, inducing first ray plantarflexion and the typical height of the medial arch.[1,2,12]

Rotatory malalignment is another classic feature of the cavo varus foot. The forefoot is consequently pushed in to hyperpronation and adduction due to the plantar fascia contraction. A similar rotatory movement acts at the Chopart joints, plantar-shifting the cuboid bone to the navicular bone.

The Chopart joint becomes locked and fixed into varus, overloading the lateral side of the foot. A combination of the consequent subtalar locking adjustment and the weakness of peroneus brevis may lead to the onset of lateral ankle instability.[1,13]

Rotational malalignment is one of the several reasons for lateral ankle instability, which correlates cavus foot and ankle pathologies.

The evolution from supple to stiff deformity plays a key role, forcing talus into a varus tilt. This final varus malalignment may lead to a medial overload and evolution into medial ankle osteoarthritis.[2,14]

CLINICAL EVALUATION

Although observed symptoms may be misleading, the patient's interview and gait observation are still important main steps.

Pain along the lateral column of the foot is the most common complaint in patients with a cavo varus foot. Sometimes patients with a varus deformity may refer to this as "ankle instability."Furthermore, varus malalignment has been identified as a source of failure for lateral ligament reconstructions.[11,15]

Clinical examination should focus on any pathologic features.

Patient observation (standing and walking) are mandatory to detect any pathologic changes. Drop-foot compensations during swing phase and extensor hallucis longus overuse are both to be investigated.

Any pathologic correlation or stiffness between hindfoot, midfoot, and forefoot should be inspected.

The Coleman block test allows the identification of a "forefoot-driven" deformity, given by an isolate first ray plantarflexion.[16]

The Silferskjöld test may be used to assess gastrocnemius-soleus complex function.

Pain and tenderness along the peroneal tendons (especially of Muscle peroneus brevis) may be investigated to plan any specific imaging studies.

The hyperactivity of the peroneus longus to selectively plantar flex the first ray should also be assessed.

Last, patients with a cavo varus foot should undergo a neurologic screening to evaluate the presence of Charct Marie Tooth or any other systemic peripheral neuropathies.

IMAGING

Weight-bearing foot and ankle radiographs are mandatory for diagnosis and treatment.[16]

A correlation between cavo varus foot and spina bifida and other spine deformities has been previously proved. We advocate to complete imaging planning with plain lumbosacral radiographs.[17,18]

Our focus is to analyze how a cavo varus foot affects the ankle.

Weight-bearing views that correlate the tibia, talus, and calcaneus are the key examinations to make any assessments on this topic. Cobey[19] described the original method which was later modified by Saltzman and el-Khoury.[20] The successful modified method reliably correlates the hindfoot and the ankle, although some authors have more recently pointed out the limits of reliability for this view.[20,21]

Modern improvements in cone-beam computed tomography now allow standing weight-bearing imaging of the lower extremity with low radiation dose. There is an increasing amount of literature describing the use of weight-bearing computed tomography in patients with foot and ankle disorders. At the moment, these studies are focusing on the qualitative advantage brought by a 3-dimensional vision; we advocate an upgrade in terms of reliability, developing specific protocols, and worldwide availability.[21,22]

An important challenge is to correlate rotational midfoot deformity (Chopart joints level) with hindfoot supination and inframalleolar deformity.

In fact, the talonavicular coverage angle is the most common tool to compare hindfoot position and forefoot abduction-adduction.[23,24] It is defined as being positive when the navicular articular axis is lateral to the talar articular axis and negative when the opposite occurs. It has been extensively used for flat foot deformities in several treatment algorithms, but it similarly may be used for the cavo varus foot deformity.[23] One limitation is the lack of any correlation with ankle inframalleolar deformities.

TREATMENT

Cavo varus foot is a multifactorial pathology. The ideal surgical treatment has to address every pathologic issue. Proper planning has to take in consideration if the deformity is supple or rigid, where is the center of rotation of angulation (CORA) of the deformity, and any muscular weakness.[21,25] More recently, the literature pointed to the strong correlation between cavo varus foot and ankle alignment.

Corrective procedures include soft tissue releases, tendon transfer, osteotomies, and fusions at different levels.

The goal is to obtain a stable, balanced, plantigrade foot and ankle complex.

Bone Procedures

Calcaneal osteotomies

Numerous techniques have been described for the correction of the hindfoot varus.

American osteotomies

One of the most popular procedures was developed by Dwyer.[26] The Dwyer osteotomy consists of a lateral oblique incision over the tuberosity of the calcaneus, a closing-wedge osteotomy, and a subsequent lateralization of the tuberosity. The main concerns are insufficient correction in the case of more severe deformity and the alteration of the Achilles-lever arm with consequent triceps weakness. An additional disadvantage is calcaneus shortening (**Fig. 1**).[3]

Probably, one of the most used calcaneus osteotomies is the lateralizing calcaneal osteotomy. This procedure requires a similar approach to the Dwyer, with a simple lateral sliding osteotomy. The principal advantage of this technique is the possible large amount of calcaneal translation. The main disadvantage is that no multiplanar correction is achievable (**Fig. 2**).[3] Furthermore, excessive lateral sliding may decrease the tarsal tunnel volume, causing neurologic symptoms.[27–29]

Another option described, but less used and advertised, is the posterior displacement osteotomy. It is designed to provide a posterior and superior shifting of the tuberosity with a lateral approach. Theoretically, it may improve the lever arm of

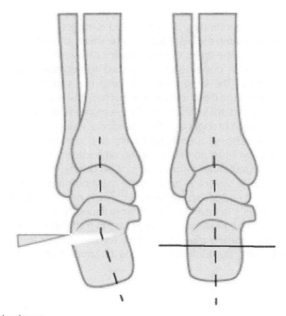

Fig. 1. Dwyer osteotomy.

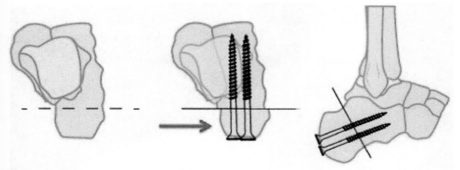

Fig. 2. Lateralizing calcaneal osteotomy.

Achilles with a functional improvement. The authors have no experience with this technique.[30]

European osteotomies

The Z-osteotomy was first described by Pisani.[31] This osteotomy was originally described as an L-shaped closing-wedge osteotomy. Pisani's goal was to design an osteotomy with a large surface of contact, strong intrinsic stability, and high potential of correction. Later, the L-osteotomy was converted into a Z-shaped osteotomy by Malerba and De Marchi,[32] adding a single further arm to the original one of Pisani.[31] Malerba and De Marchi[32] described a closing-wedge lateral-based Z-shaped osteotomy, with no translation of the tuberosity. The advantage reported was an improvement of the contact between the bone resections, without supporting any displacements. Despite this, the Z-osteotomy has been popularized as the most powerful correction for the hindfoot varus. Other investigators, more recently, claimed that this procedure, as originally described, would not allow a larger correction than L-shaped and previous different osteotomies.

Hintermann and colleagues[33] improved this Z-osteotomy, describing a rotation of the tuberosity and dorsal lengthening when necessary. This modified osteotomy really allowed powerful triplanar correction, finally. It can be a challenging osteotomy technique, due to the complexity of the osteotomy cuts and unintentional overcorrection has been described (**Figs. 3** and **4**).[34]

Fusions

This article is focused on calcaneal osteotomies. However, corrective bony cuts are contraindicated in the case of stiff arthritic deformity. In similar conditions, fusion should be the advisable option.

Arthrodesis has been previously described through every segment of the foot.

Isolateral subtalar joint fusion, hindfoot double arthrodesis through the talonavicular and calcaneal–cuboid joints, and triple fusion are powerful and predictable procedures for multiplanar cavus foot correction. The primary goal is to achieve a proper alignment of the foot and ankle complex. The ideal consequence is to obtain a balanced, well-aligned ankle and prevent the onset of ankle arthritis.[35]

In any kind of hindfoot deformities, lateral column length is a critical topic.

Calcaneo-cuboid joint is the key to act at the CORA of the deformity, both for the cavo varus foot (with forefoot adduction) and for the valgus flat foot (with forefoot abduction).[2]

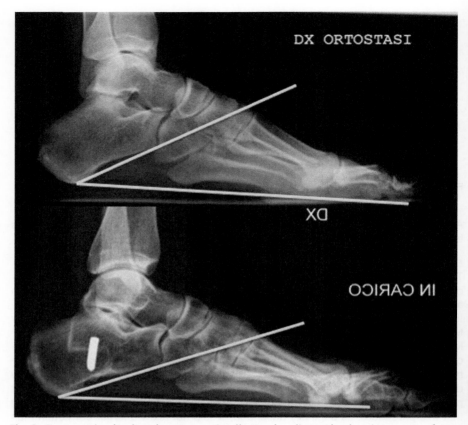

Fig. 3. Preoperative (*top*) and postoperative (*bottom*) radiographs showing a case of cavo varus deformity (2-A2 according to our classification) treated with Z-shaped calcaneal osteotomy.

Isolateral shortening of the calcaneo-cuboidal arthrodesis has been proposed as a very efficient tool in those deformities with an important adduction moment. It benefits from possessing a great potential for correction, without a relevant loss of function. Further assessments are required to measure the real impact of this procedure on an ankle inframalleolar deformities.[35,36]

TRANSFER

Soft tissue release, osteotomy, and fusion procedures require appropriate muscular balancing, otherwise they are doomed to fail.

Different patterns of dysfunction may require different tendon transfer procedures. The proper treatment should be designed according to a deep understanding of the pathology and requires a bone procedure to correct the deformity.[37]

Several patterns of muscle imbalance have been described for the cavo varus foot, but they can basically be divided into 2 groups.

The first is due to an overpowered posterior tibial tendon and the concomitant peroneus brevis weakness. This mechanism induces foot inversion.

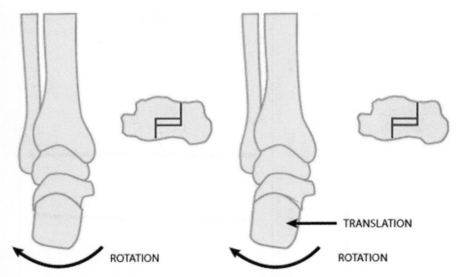

Fig. 4. Z-shaped calcaneal osteotomy for 3-plane correction.

The second is linked to the anterior tibial muscle weakness. It is responsible for different levels of drop-foot and consequent cock-up hallux deformity.

Peroneus longus to brevis transfer addresses the first described pattern. It reduces the plantarflexion moment of the medial column and inversion of the whole foot. In the early stages of a supple cavo varus foot, it adequately compensates for the dysfunction.[37,38]

Severe inversion deformity combined with drop-foot dysfunction may be treated with a posterior tibial tendon transfer on either the lateral cuneiform or the cuboid.

As previously explained, extensor hallucis and extensor digitorum muscles are recruited to improve dorsiflexion to the ankle in case of anterior tibialis weakness. This is the pathomechanic mechanism for the cock-up hallux deformity. The Jones procedure addresses this phenomenon with an extensor hallux longus transfer to the first metatarsal neck and the fusion of hallux interphalangeal joint.[37]

DISCUSSION

Cavo varus foot deformities are always a difficult challenge for physicians. Subtle neurologic dysfunctions may be suspected, even in patients with a negative neurologic screening.[39]

Joint-preserving surgery is the main goal, especially in young and active patients. It requires a combination of bone and soft tissue procedures. The ideal treatment should address both deformity correction and deforming forces neutralization.

Patients must be aware that the cavo varus foot is a progressive rather than a static pathology and further surgeries may be necessary in the future.[40]

Undercorrection is the main issue when dealing with the cavo varus foot deformity, especially on long-term follow-up.

Our explanation focuses on 2 different reasons: evolution of the pathology (linked to the single patient's features and pathology evolution) and understanding of the deformity (linked to the physician's treatment algorithm).

Table 1
Algorithm of treatment for cavo varus foot

Stage	Substage	Clinical Findings	Radiographic Findings	Hindfoot Alignment	Forefoot Adduction	Ankle Alignment	Forefoot Alignment	HF-Ankle Mechanical Axis	Procedures
I	A	Normal anatomy Tenderness along peroneal tendons	Normal anatomy	Neutral	No	Neutral			NSAIDs Cryotherapy Physical Therapy Tendoscopy
	B	Slight HF varus Tenderness along peroneal tendons	Slight HF varus	Neutral-slightly varus	No	Neutral			NSAIDs Cryotherapy Physical Therapy Orthoses Tendoscopy

II							
A1	Coleman block test + Supple HF varus	*1st metatarsal plantarflexion* Meary line disruption Calcaneal pitch angle increase HF varus	Varus	No	Neutral or moderate varus		*1st metatarsal dorsiflexion osteotomy* + tendon transfers ("a-la-carte")
A2	Coleman block test - Supple HF varus	*1st metatarsal plantarflexion (inconstant finding)* Meary line disruption Calcaneal pitch angle increase HF varus	Varus	No	Neutral or moderate varus		*1st metatarsal dorsiflexion osteotomy (if necessary)* + calcaneal osteotomy + tendon transfers ("a-la-carte")

(continued on next page)

Table 1
(continued)

Stage	Substage	Clinical Findings	Radiographic Findings	Hindfoot Alignment	Forefoot Adduction	Ankle Alignment	Forefoot Alignment	HF-Ankle Mechanical Axis	Procedures
	B1	Forefoot adduction Supple HF varus	Talonavicular overcoverage HF varus	Varus	Yes	Neutral or moderate varus + Slightly Intrarotation			CC joint fusion (shortening) + tendon transfers ("a-la-carte")
	B2	*1st ray plantarflexion* Forefoot adduction Supple HF varus	*1st metatarsal plantarflexion* Talonavicular overcoverage HF varus	Varus	Yes	Neutral or moderate varus + Slightly Intrarotation			*1st metatarsal dorsiflexion* osteotomy + CC joint fusion (shortening) + tendon transfers ("a-la-carte")

III	A	*Fixed forefoot pronation* Rigid HF varus Painful subtalar joint	*1st metatarsal plantarflexion* HF varus Subtalar joint space loss	Varus	No	Neutral or moderate varus		*Midfoot dorsiflexion osteotomy or fusion* + ST joint fusion + tendon transfers ("a-la-carte")
	B	*Fixed forefoot pronation* Forefoot adduction Rigid HF varus Painful subtalar joint	*1st metatarsal plantarflexion* Talonavicular overcoverage HF varus Subtalar joint space loss	Varus	Yes	Neutral or moderate varus + Slightly Intrarotation		ST joint fusion + CC joint fusion (shortening) + midfoot dorsiflexion osteotomy or fusion + tendon transfers ("a-la-carte")

(continued on next page)

Table 1
(continued)

Stage	Substage	Clinical Findings	Radiographic Findings	Hindfoot Alignment	Forefoot Adduction	Ankle Alignment	Forefoot Alignment Axis	HF-Ankle Mechanical Axis	Procedures
IV	A1	Supple lower limb varus (below the knee)	Tibiotalar varus HF varus	Varus	No	Severe varus			SMOT (when indicated) Surgery for HF varus + tendon transfers ("a-la-carte") **(Fig. 6)**
	A2	Supple lower limb varus (below the knee) Forefoot adduction	Tibiotalar varus HF varus Talonavicular overcoverage	Varus	Yes	Varus + intrarotation			SMOT (when indicated) + CC joint fusion (shortening) + tendon transfers ("a-la-carte")
	A3	Supple valgus ankle with lower limb apparently aligned	Tibiotalar valgus HF varus *(ping-pong deformity)*	Varus	No	Valgus			SMOT (when indicated) HF varus correction (only if necessary after ankle correction) + deltoid reconstruction + tendon transfers ("a-la-carte")

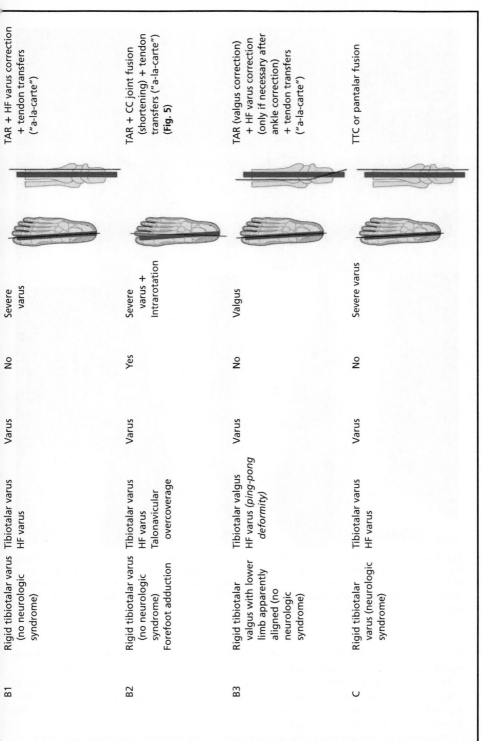

B1	Rigid tibiotalar varus (no neurologic syndrome)	Tibiotalar varus HF varus	Varus	No	Severe varus		TAR + HF varus correction + tendon transfers ("a-la-carte")
B2	Rigid tibiotalar varus (no neurologic syndrome) Forefoot adduction	Tibiotalar varus HF varus Talonavicular overcoverage	Varus	Yes	Severe varus + Intrarotation		TAR + CC joint fusion (shortening) + tendon transfers ("a-la-carte") (Fig. 5)
B3	Rigid tibiotalar valgus with lower limb apparently aligned (no neurologic syndrome)	Tibiotalar valgus HF varus (ping-pong deformity)	Varus	No	Valgus		TAR (valgus correction) + HF varus correction (only if necessary after ankle correction) + tendon transfers ("a-la-carte")
C	Rigid tibiotalar varus (neurologic syndrome)	Tibiotalar varus HF varus	Varus	No	Severe varus		TTC or pantalar fusion

Green describes the physiologic range of the mechanical axis, black describes the ideal mechanical axis, red defines the pathologic mechanical axis.

Abbreviations: CC, calcaneocuboid; HF, hindfoot; SMOT, supramalleolar osteotomy; ST, subtalar; TAR, total ankle replacement; TTC, tibio talar calcaneus (fusion).

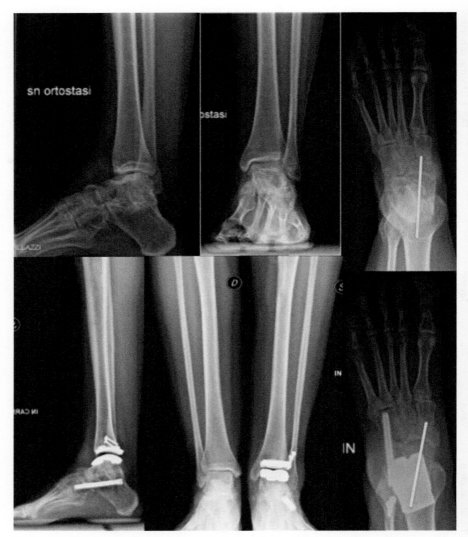

Fig. 5. Preoperative and postoperative radiographs showing a case of inframalleolar rotational deformity related to forefoot adduction (4-2B according to our classification). Forefoot adduction was addressed with calcaneocuboid joint fusion (shortening), inframalleolar deformity was addressed with shortening and de-rotational fibula osteotomy + total ankle replacement.

Several biomechanics theories have been proposed, but the development of a treatment algorithm is still challenging due to the heterogeneity of the pathology.[41]

Historically, Pisani[42] first introduced the concept of a hindfoot-complex instability in the cavo varus foot with the principle of "coxa pedis." This definition refers to the talar-navicular and anterior subtalar joints, comparing their shape and function to the femoral head into the acetabular pavement.[42,43]

"Coxa pedis" turned out to be a predictive model to study the cavo varus foot.

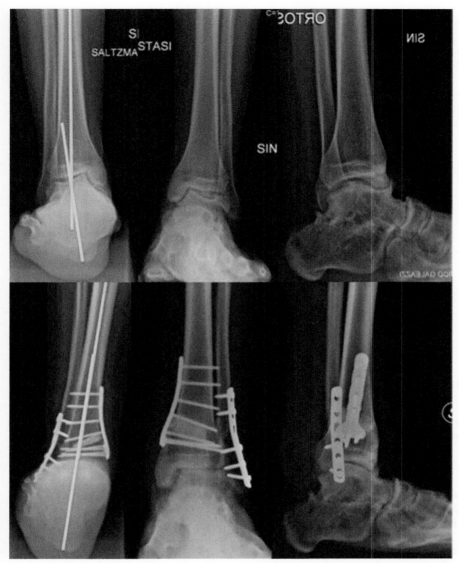

Fig. 6. Preoperative (*top*) and postoperative (*bottom*) radiographs of a case of varus ankle deformity (4-A1 according to our classification). The patient was previously treated with a hindfoot procedure (calcaneal osteotomy and subtalar joint fusion) in another hospital. The correction was not powerful enough because the apex of the deformity is in the ankle. According to our algorithm, we treated the patient with supramalleolar osteotomy.

However, the theory, as originally described, did not yet focus on ankle instability and inframalleolar deformity. Hintermann and colleagues[43] later developed this topic with the definition of "peritalar instability."

Our group has recently proposed a novel classification linking ankle instability to ankle and hindfoot ("coxa pedis") varus deformities. We stratified lateral peritalar

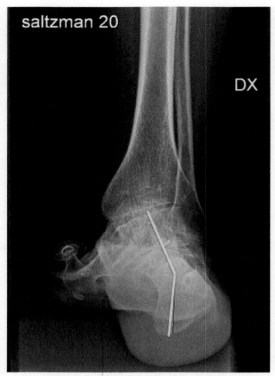

Fig. 7. Ping-pong deformity: valgus arthritic ankle in combination with a cavo varus foot.

instability in 3 different groups: axis deviation, ligamentous instability, and functional instability.[10]

However, this classification does not focus on the analysis of the cavo varus foot deformity. A second limitation is the lack of a clear algorithm of treatment.

A scientific approach to this pathology would require a comprehensive classification and an algorithm of treatment to clearly select those patients who would benefit from calcaneal osteotomies not only for hindfoot, but for inframalleolar deformities correction as well.[44–46]

The main author (FGU) discloses his own daily algorithm of treatment for cavo varus foot in **Table 1**.

Calcaneal osteotomies exceed their primary goal to exclusively correct varus heel deformities. They may have a role as part of a treatment for moderate varus hindfoot and ankle deformity corrections.[2] As previously stated by Hintermann and colleagues,[45] all calcaneal osteotomies have limited power to correct at the ankle level and, in the case of severe ankle deformity, it is advisable to plan proximal corrections.

Hindfoot Varus Ankle Valgus: Ping-Pong Deformity

Some patterns of deformities may be more challenging than what is presumable at the initial assessment. Ankle valgus is not always correlated with pronated flat foot deformity. Indeed, valgus ankle may underlie a cavo varus foot. The key problem is deltoid insufficiency that may occur as a consequence of a multidirectional instability, given by prolonged chronic lateral ligament incompetence. The resulting chronic medial instability overloads the posterior lateral aspect of the tibial plafond with gradual erosion and subsequent talar valgus deformity. The obvious endpoint is the onset of a valgus arthritic ankle in combination with a cavo varus foot. This phenomenon has been previously described as a ping-pong deformity (**Fig. 7**).[47–49]

In these cases, the senior author (FGU) recommends to plan valgus correction in the ankle (bone and soft tissue reconstruction) first and rely on calcaneal osteotomies only in the case of a residual deformity at the end of the surgery.

SUMMARY

The cavo varus foot is a challenging deformity.

The calcaneal osteotomy has a role in the correction of hindfoot deformities and consequent moderate inframalleolar deformities.

Although several calcaneal osteotomies with a high power of correction have been proposed, rigorous weight-bearing imaging planning is still key to avoid underestimating ankle deformities and rotational foot deformities that cannot be addressed by iso-lateral calcaneal osteotomies.

ACKNOWLEDGMENTS

Our sincerest thanks go to Dr Camilla Maccario for her support in developing this paper.

REFERENCES

1. Aminian A, Sangeorzan BJ. The anatomy of cavus foot deformity. Foot Ankle Clin 2008;13(2):191–8, v.
2. Klaue K. Hindfoot issues in the treatment of the cavovarus foot. Foot Ankle Clin 2008;13(2):221–7, vi.
3. Bariteau JT, Blankenhorn BD, Tofte JN, et al. What is the role and limit of calcaneal osteotomy in the cavovarus foot? Foot Ankle Clin 2013;18(4):697–714.
4. Manoli A 2nd, Graham B. The subtle cavus foot, "the underpronator" [review]. Foot Ankle Int 2005;26(3):256–63.
5. Knupp M, Stufkens SA, Bolliger L, et al. Classification and treatment of supramalleolar deformities. Foot Ankle Int 2011;32(11):1023–31.
6. Hintermann B, Knupp M, Barg A. Joint-preserving surgery of asymmetric ankle osteoarthritis with peritalar instability. Foot Ankle Clin 2013;18(3):503–16.
7. Tallroth K, Harilainen A, Kerttula L, et al. Ankle osteoarthritis is associated with knee osteoarthritis. Conclusions based on mechanical axis radiographs. Arch Orthop Trauma Surg 2008;128(6):555–60.
8. Richter M, Zech S. Lengthening osteotomy of the calcaneus and flexor digitorum longus tendon transfer in flexible flat foot deformity improves talo-1st metatarsal-Index, clinical outcome and pedographic parameter. Foot Ankle Surg 2013;19(1):56–61.
9. Bluman EM, Title CI, Myerson MS. Posterior tibial tendon rupture: a refined classification system [review]. Foot Ankle Clin 2007;12(2):233–49, v.
10. Usuelli FG, Mason L, Grassi M, et al. Lateral ankle and hindfoot instability: a new clinical based classification. Foot Ankle Surg 2014;20(4):231–6.
11. Klammer G, Benninger E, Espinosa N. The varus ankle and instability. Foot Ankle Clin 2012;17(1):57–82.

12. Usuelli FG, D'Ambrosi R, Manzi L, et al. Clinical outcomes and return to sports in patients with chronic Achilles tendon rupture after minimally invasive reconstruction with semitendinosus tendon graft transfer. Joints 2017;5(4):212–6.

13. Pagenstert GI, Hintermann B, Barg A, et al. Realignment surgery as alternative treatment of varus and valgus ankle osteoarthritis. Clin Orthop Relat Res 2007; 462:156–68.

14. Valderrabano V, Horisberger M, Russell I, et al. Etiology of ankle osteoarthritis. Clin Orthop Relat Res 2009;467(7):1800–6.

15. Strauss JE, Forsberg JA, Lippert FG 3rd. Chronic lateral ankle instability and associated conditions: a rationale for treatment. Foot Ankle Int 2007;28(10): 1041–4.

16. Perera A, Guha A. Clinical and radiographic evaluation of the cavus foot: surgical implications. Foot Ankle Clin 2013;18(4):619–28.

17. Berjano P, Lamartina C. Classification of degenerative segment disease in adults with deformity of the lumbar or thoracolumbar spine. Eur Spine J 2014;23(9): 1815–24.

18. Garbossa D, Pejrona M, Damilano M, et al. Pelvic parameters and global spine balance for spine degenerative disease: the importance of containing for the well being of content. Eur Spine J 2014;23(Suppl 6):616–27.

19. Cobey JC. Posterior roentgenogram of the foot. Clin Orthop Relat Res 1976;118: 202–7.

20. Saltzman CL, el-Khoury GY. The hindfoot alignment view. Foot Ankle Int 1995; 16(9):572–6.

21. Nosewicz TL, Knupp M, Bolliger L, et al. The reliability and validity of radiographic measurements for determining the three-dimensional position of the talus in varus and valgus osteoarthritic ankles. Skeletal Radiol 2012;41(12):1567–73.

22. Barg A, Bailey T, Richter M, et al. Weightbearing computed tomography of the foot and ankle: emerging technology topical review. Foot Ankle Int 2018;39(3): 376–86.

23. Ellis SJ, Yu JC, Williams BR, et al. New radiographic parameters assessing forefoot abduction in the adult acquired flatfoot deformity. Foot Ankle Int 2009;30: 1168–76.

24. Paley D, Lamm BM. Correction of the cavus foot using external fixation. Foot Ankle Clin 2004 Sep;9(3):611–24, x.

25. Myerson MS. Cavus foot correction. In: Myerson MS, editor. Reconstructive foot and ankle surgery. Philadelphia: Elsevier Saunders; 2005. p. 153–68.

26. Dwyer FC. Osteotomy of the calcaneum for pes cavus. J Bone Joint Surg Br 1959;41:80–6.

27. Cody EA, Greditzer HG 4th, MacMahon A, et al. Effects on the tarsal tunnel following malerba Z-type osteotomy compared to standard lateralizing calcaneal osteotomy. Foot Ankle Int 2016;37(9):1017–22.

28. Bruce BG, Bariteau JT, Evangelista PE, et al. The effect of medial and lateral calcaneal osteotomies on the tarsal tunnel. Foot Ankle Int 2014;35(4):383–8.

29. Krause FG, Pohl MJ, Penner MJ, et al. Tibial nerve palsy associated with lateralizing calcaneal osteotomy: case reviews and technical tip. Foot Ankle Int 2009; 30(3):258–61.

30. Mitchell GP. Posterior displacement osteotomy of the calcaneus. J Bone Joint Surg Br 1977;59(2):233–5.

31. Pisani G. Osteotomie sous-talamique par la correction chirurgicale des deformations du calcaneum dans le plan frontal (varus, valgus) [Subtalar osteotomy for

correction of deformities of the calcaneus in the frontal plane]. In: Podologie. Paris (France); 1985.

32. Malerba F, De Marchi F. Calcaneal osteotomies. Foot Ankle Clin 2005;10: 523–40, vii.

33. Knupp M, Horisberger M, Hintermann B. A new Z-shaped calcaneal osteotomy for 3-plane correction of severe varus deformity of the hindfoot. Tech Foot Ankle Surg 2008;7(2):90–5.

34. Vermeulen K, Neven E, Vandeputte G, et al. Relationship of the scarf valgus-inducing osteotomy of the calcaneus to the medial neurovascular structures. Foot Ankle Int 2011;32(5):S540–4.

35. Zide JR, Myerson MS. Arthrodesis for the cavus foot: when, where, and how? Foot Ankle Clin 2013;18(4):755–67.

36. Seringe R. Congenital equinovarus clubfoot. Acta Orthop Belg 1999;65(2): 127–53.

37. Huber M. What is the role of tendon transfer in the cavus foot? Foot Ankle Clin 2013;18(4):689–95.

38. Guelfi M, Pantalone A, Mirapeix RM, et al. Anatomy, pathophysiology and classification of posterior tibial tendon dysfunction. Eur Rev Med Pharmacol Sci 2017; 21(1):13–9.

39. Tuinhout M, Anderson PG, Louwerens JW. Foot Build Registration System (FBRS) to evaluate foot posture: a reliability study with healthy subjects and patients with Charcot-Marie-Tooth disease. Foot Ankle Surg 2009;15(3):127–32.

40. Guyton GP, Mann RA. The pathogenesis and surgical management of foot deformity in Charcot-Marie-Tooth disease [review]. Foot Ankle Clin 2000;5(2):317–26.

41. Moraleda L, Mubarak SJ. Flexible flatfoot: differences in the relative alignment of each segment of the foot between symptomatic and asymptomatic patients. J Pediatr Orthop 2011;31:421–8.

42. Pisani G. "Coxa pedis" today. Foot Ankle Surg 2016;22(2):78–84.

43. Hintermann B, Knupp M, Barg A. Peritalar instability. Foot Ankle Int 2012;33(5): 450–4.

44. Hintermann B, Valderrabano V, Kundert HP. Lengthening of the lateral column and reconstruction of the medial soft tissue for treatment of acquired flatfoot deformity associated with insufficiency of the posterior tibial tendon. Foot Ankle Int 1999;20(10):622–9.

45. Hintermann B, Ruiz R, Barg A. Novel double osteotomy technique of distal tibia for correction of asymmetric varus osteoarthritic ankle. Foot Ankle Int 2017; 38(9):970–81.

46. Louie PK, Sangeorzan BJ, Fassbind MJ, et al. Talonavicular joint coverage and bone morphology between different foot types. J Orthop Res 2014;32(7):958–66.

47. Dodd A, Daniels TR. Total ankle replacement in the presence of talar varus or valgus deformities. Foot Ankle Clin 2017;22(2):277–300.

48. Usuelli FG, Maccario C, Manzi L, et al. Clinical outcome and fusion rate following simultaneous subtalar fusion and total ankle arthroplasty. Foot Ankle Int 2016; 37(7):696–702.

49. Krause F, Windolf M, Schweiger K, et al. Ankle joint pressure in pes cavovarus. J Bone Joint Surg Br 2007;89:1660–5.

Joint-Preserving Procedures in Patients with Varus Deformity
Role of Supramalleolar Osteotomies

Alexej Barg, MD*, Charles L. Saltzman, MD*

KEYWORDS

- Tibiotalar joint • Varus tibiotalar osteoarthritis • Supramalleolar varus deformity
- Medial opening-wedge supramalleolar osteotomy
- Lateral closing-wedge supramalleolar osteotomy

KEY POINTS

- The most common cause for end-stage ankle osteoarthritis is posttraumatic, often resulting in concomitant supramalleolar deformity.
- Aims of the supramalleolar osteotomy include restoration of the lower-leg axis to improve intraarticular load distribution, retard degeneration of the tibiotalar joint, and improve function.
- Preoperative planning is based on conventional weight-bearing radiographs. Often advanced imaging, including computed tomography and/or MRI, can help clarify the underlying problem and potentially allow for a supramalleolar correction.
- For a varus deformity, a supramalleolar osteotomy can be corrected either through the medial approach with a medial opening-wedge osteotomy or through the lateral approach with a lateral closing-wedge osteotomy.
- Complete pain relief should not be expected following a supramalleolar osteotomy procedure. Postoperative complications are not uncommon, including progression of tibiotalar osteoarthritis.

INTRODUCTION

The most common cause for end-stage ankle osteoarthritis (OA) is posttraumatic, accounting for 80% of all cases[1,2] and most commonly following lower-leg fractures[3,4] and/or repetitive ankle sprains.[5] Therefore, it is not surprising that patients with

Department of Orthopaedics, University of Utah, 590 Wakara Way, Salt Lake City, UT 84108, USA
* Corresponding authors.
E-mail addresses: alexej.barg@hsc.utah.edu (A.B.); charles.saltzman@hsc.utah.edu (C.L.S.)

Foot Ankle Clin N Am 24 (2019) 239–264
https://doi.org/10.1016/j.fcl.2019.02.004
1083-7515/19/© 2019 Elsevier Inc. All rights reserved.
foot.theclinics.com

Table 1
Radiographic hindfoot alignment in the coronal plane in patients with end-stage ankle osteoarthritis: posttraumatic (166 ankles) versus primary (13 ankle) versus rheumatoid (17 ankles) osteoarthritis

Parameter	Patients with Posttraumatic OA	Patients with Primary OA	Patients with Rheumatoid OA	P Value
Gender, male: female	89:77	7:6	4:13	.060[c]
Age (y)	56.7 ± 14.1 (18–85)	67.4 ± 6.9 (54–75)	58.9 ± 13.0 (30–75)	.024[d]
Medial distal tibial angle (°)	85.9 ± 7.1 (66.3–123.7)	85.6 ± 6.2 (75.0–96.7)	89.0 ± 5.2 (83.3–102.0)	.206[d]
Tibiotalar surface angle (°)	82.9 ± 13.1 (45.3–122.7)	85.5 ± 15.6 (64.0–115.3)	85.3 ± 14.9 (60.7–111.0)	.636[d]
Talar tilting angle (°)[a]	−3.0 ± 11.6 (−41.3–28.7)	−0.1 ± 13.9 (−17.0–28.0)	−3.7 ± 12.5 (−25.3–17.0)	.656[d]
Tibiocalcaneal axis angle (°)[a]	−9.7 ± 10.9 (−47.3–20.3)	−3.9 ± 6.8 (−13.3–9.0)	0.8 ± 16.5 (−22.3–25.3)	.001[d]
Moment arm of calcaneus (mm)[b]	−6.5 ± 18.1 (−88.7–39.2)	−8.4 ± 13.2 (−15.2–22.1)	4.1 ± 22.0 (−42.6–37.5)	.048[d]

[a] Negative values indicate varus malalignment.
[b] Negative values indicate the lowest point of the calcaneus was medial to the longitudinal axis of the tibia (varus malalignment).
[c] Using χ^2 test.
[d] Using ANOVA (analysis of variance test).
    Data from Wang B, Saltzman CL, Chalayon O, et al. Does the subtalar joint compensate for ankle malalignment in end-stage ankle arthritis? Clin Orthop Relat Res 2015;473(1):318–25.

end-stage ankle OA often present with a concomitant deformity that may be seen at the supramalleolar, intraarticular, and/or inframalleolar level.[3,6] Wang and colleagues[7] analyzed radiographs of 226 patients (233 ankles) with end-stage symptomatic ankle OA (**Table 1**). Perfect alignment with ankle OA is rare. Indeed, 27.5% had supramalleolar varus deformity, 8.2% had supramalleolar valgus deformity, and only 64.4% were within 2 standard deviations of the normal population (**Fig. 1**).[7] At the inframalleolar level, 21.9% had varus deformity, 18.9% had valgus deformity, and only 59.2% had inframalleolar alignment within 2 standard deviations of the normal population (see **Fig. 1**).[7] In patients with a concomitant supramalleolar deformity, an asymmetric joint load can be expected,[8,9] which may result in asymmetric cartilage damage with a partially preserved tibiotalar joint.[10,11]

In 1936, Speed and Boyd[12] first described realignment surgery in patients with malunited fractures about the ankle joint. The investigators stated the following 3 aims of the reconstruction operation[12]:

1. Restoration of the proper weight-bearing alignment of the leg as a whole;
2. Restoration of the normal anatomic relationship between the articular surfaces of the tibia and the astragalus;
3. Restoration of a satisfactory range of painless motion.

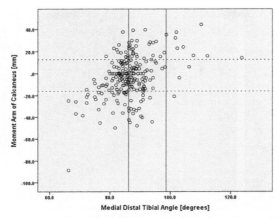

Fig. 1. Supramalleolar and inframalleolar alignment in 233 patients with end-stage ankle OA. Two vertical lines indicate a range of 2 standard deviations for the medial distal tibial angle (83.3° to 94.9°). Two horizontal dashed lines indicate a range of 2 standard deviations for the moment arm of calcaneus (−16.6–14.2 mm). Negative values indicate that the lowest point of the calcaneus was medial to the longitudinal axis line of the tibia (varus alignment).

Eighty years later, the aims of supramalleolar osteotomy (SMOT) remain the same: restoration of the lower-leg axis to improve intraarticular load distribution and consequently slow down or even stop degeneration of the tibiotalar joint.[13–25] This article highlights the use of supramalleolar osteotomies in patients with varus ankle OA.

INDICATIONS AND CONTRAINDICATIONS FOR SUPRAMALLEOLAR OSTEOTOMY

The most common indication for SMOT is the *supramalleolar* varus deformity with a partially preserved tibiotalar joint on the central and lateral aspects. In patients with end-stage ankle OA requiring total ankle replacement or ankle arthrodesis, SMOT may help improve the overall lower-leg axis and achieve optimal postoperative outcomes. Several studies have demonstrated that unaddressed malalignment may negatively influence clinical outcomes, especially in patients who have undergone total ankle replacement.[26–29]

The contraindications for supramalleolar osteotomies can be divided into general and procedure-specific contraindications. The general contraindications include acute or chronic infection with or without osteomyelitis, severe vascular or neurologic deficiency, or neuropathic disorders (eg, Charcot arthropathy).[30] Patients with end-stage varus OA that affects the entire tibiotalar joint, including medial, central, and lateral compartments, should undergo total ankle replacement or ankle arthrodesis. This contraindication is discussed in other articles in this issue. Another specific contraindication for this procedure is patients' noncompliance; rehabilitation is long and complex and requires absolute non-weight-bearing for several weeks. Finally, the SMOT should not be recommended to patients with unrealistic expectations. Complete pain relief after realignment surgery is unlikely (see **Table 5**),[31–37] and the complete recovery process often takes several years. The patient must fully understand that if pain relief is inadequate after a sufficient period of time, a joint-removing surgery (replacement, arthrodesis) may be needed.

In addition to monitoring for absolute contraindications, all relative contraindications should be carefully considered. Performing supramalleolar osteotomies on patients with relative contraindications may result in a higher rate of complications and worse

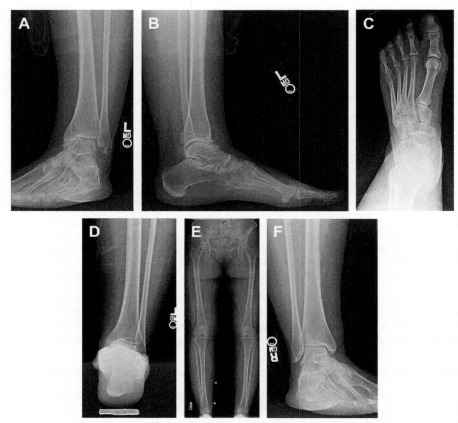

Fig. 2. Weight-bearing conventional radiographs of a 45-year-old female patient with post-traumatic ligamentous tibiotalar OA. (*A*) Mortise view of the ankle. (*B*) Lateral and (*C*) dorsoplantar views of the foot. (*D*) Hindfoot alignment view. A medial distal tibial angle of 84°, a tibiotalar tilt of 6° varus, and a calcaneal moment arm of 19 mm varus. (*E*) Whole-leg radiograph. (*F*) Mortise view of the contralateral healthy ankle for comparison.

clinical outcomes.[30] Supramalleolar osteotomies are relatively contraindicated in patients with substantially impaired bone quality, such as patients with long-term steroid medication, severe osteoporosis, and rheumatoid disease. Uncontrolled diabetes is another relative contraindication for this type of surgery because it may result in a higher rate of perioperative (eg, wound-healing problems) or postoperative (eg, osteotomy nonunion) complications.[38,39] Frailty is another relative contraindication, because the recovery period is long, and these patients are often best served by a single definitive procedure. However, the current literature has no clear recommendation on the age limit for this surgery.[30] Finally, tobacco use is a relative contraindication because nicotine may negatively influence osseous healing.[40]

PREOPERATIVE PLANNING

For preoperative radiographic assessment, the authors routinely recommend the use of conventional weight-bearing radiographs, including 4 standardized views: lateral and dorsoplantar views of the foot, mortise view of the ankle, and hindfoot alignment view (**Fig. 2**).[41,42] In addition, whole-leg radiographs are crucial to assess the osseous deformities of the entire lower extremity (see **Fig. 2**). It has been demonstrated that some patients may have both a knee and ankle pathologic condition with some compensatory alignment changes occurring at each joint.[43] For a more comprehensive assessment, the authors also recommend bilateral weight-bearing radiographs (see **Fig. 2**). Recently, Haraguchi and colleagues[44] described the novel hip-to-calcaneus radiographs used for preoperative and postoperative radiographic assessment in patients who underwent a SMOT for varus ankle OA (**Fig. 3**). Conventional whole-leg radiographs traditionally identify the mechanical axis with a line positioned from the center of the femoral head to the center of the tibial plafond.[45] This traditional assessment of the mechanical axis ignores the alignment underneath the tibiotalar joint, the inframalleolar alignment, and its effect on overall alignment. The Haraguchi method allows for exact alignment of the lower-leg axis from the hip to the calcaneus.[44]

For better assessment of degenerative changes in the tibiotalar and adjacent joints, a computed tomography (CT) scan or a weight-bearing CT (WBCT) scan should be performed. WBCT scans offer several advantages over traditional radiographs, including physiologic standing position (assessment of osseous alignment and possibly impingement), high spatial resolution (exact assessment of arthritic changes), fast imaging acquisition time (patients' convenience), and a relatively low radiation dose (lower than conventional CT scan → 0.01–0.03 mSv vs 0.07 mSv) (**Fig. 4**).[46]

The following parameters should be used for quantitative assessment of the varus deformity in the coronal plane: the medial distal tibial angle, the tibiotalar tilt, and the calcaneal moment arm (**Fig. 5**). The medial distal tibial angle is crucial for quantifying the supramalleolar varus deformity (**Table 2**). The weight-bearing mortise view of the ankle should be used for measurement of the medial distal tibial angle.[47] Measurements of this angle have been demonstrated to depend on ankle position and radiographic technique.[48,49]

Talar tilt should be used for quantitative assessment of an intraarticular deformity in the coronal plane. Viewed from the weight-bearing mortise view of the ankle, talar tilt is defined as the difference between the medial distal tibial angle and the tibiotalar angle. Values of more than 4° are considered to be pathologic (**Table 3**).[8,60]

The hindfoot alignment view should be used for quantitative assessment of an inframalleolar deformity in the coronal plane (**Table 4**).[41,42] Different measurement techniques have been described in the current literature (**Fig. 6**), including calcaneal moment arm (defined as the distance or angle between the longitudinal tibial axis and the lowest point of tuber calcanei),[42] the angle between the longitudinal tibial axis and calcaneal/subtalar joint axis,[61] and the angles between the longitudinal tibial axis and the osseous medial and lateral contours of the calcaneus.[62]

For preoperatively calculating the needed degree of correction, the authors recommend the following calculation to determine the required amount of widening or closing of the osteotomy: $H = \tan \alpha_1 \times W$, where H is the height of the wedge, α_1 is the amount of deformity, including approximately 2° of desired overcorrection, and W is the width of the distal tibia.[14,30,63,64]

SURGICAL TECHNIQUE

Both general and regional anesthesia can be used for the surgery. The patient is placed supine on the operating table. The ipsilateral pelvis is lifted to correct for the external rotation positioning of the foot. Esmarch exsanguination and a thigh tourniquet can be applied unless contraindicated. If planned, anterior ankle arthroscopy is performed using standard anterolateral and anteromedial portals.[65,66] If present,

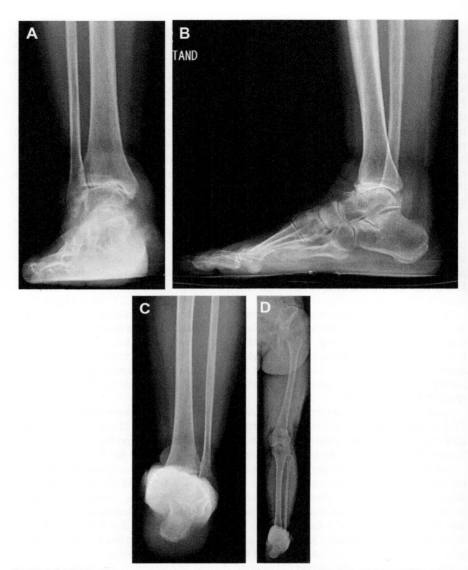

Fig. 3. Weight-bearing conventional radiographs of a 52-year-old female patient with posttraumatic ligamentous tibiotalar OA. (*A*) Mortise view of the ankle. (*B*) Lateral view of the foot. (*C*) Hindfoot alignment view. (*D*) Novel weight-bearing whole-leg hip-to-calcaneus view. (*Courtesy of* Professor Woo-Chen Lee, MD, Seoul Foot & Ankle Center, Seoul, South Korea.)

cartilage degeneration is documented and assessed using the Outerbridge classification.[67] The authors recommend intraarticular debridement of scar tissue and tenosynovitis. All osteochondral lesions encountered should be debrided with microfracturing of the exposed subchondral bone.

Supramalleolar Medial Opening-Wedge Osteotomy

A medial approach is made with a skin incision over the distal tibia and the medial malleolus. Alternatively, an anterior ankle approach can be chosen (**Fig. 7**). In patients with

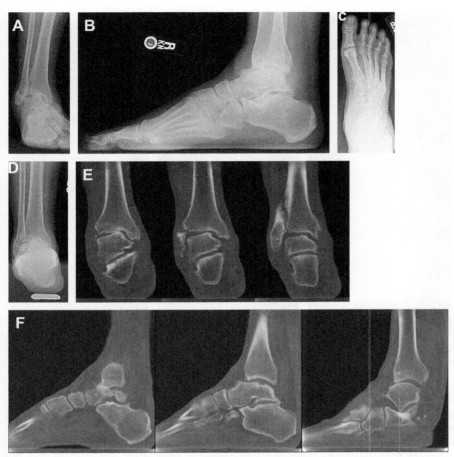

Fig. 4. Weight-bearing conventional radiographs of a 58-year-old male patient with post-traumatic ligamentous tibiotalar OA. (*A*) Mortise view of the ankle. (*B*) Lateral and (*C*) dorsoplantar views of the foot. (*D*) Hindfoot alignment view. A medial distal tibial angle of 84°, a tibiotalar tilt of 16° varus, and a calcaneal moment arm of 42 mm varus. WBCT scan, including (*E*) coronal and (*F*) sagittal slides, demonstrates varus tibiotalar OA with a partially preserved lateral compartment, a severe varus tilt, and an anterior subluxation of the talus.

previous ankle surgeries (eg, open reduction and internal fixation), an old incision or incisions should be used. If a new incision is planned, distance from the previous incision should be considered in order to avoid wound-healing problems. After the skin incision is complete, blunt dissection of the subcutaneous tissues is performed with special attention paid to not injure neurovascular structures. A subsequent incision of the periosteum exposes the distal medial tibia. The plane of the osteotomy is determined using fluoroscopy. Two horizontal Kirschner wires are placed along the osteotomy plane. As the next step, 2 Hohmann retractors are placed anteriorly and posteriorly to the distal tibia to protect the neurovascular and tendon structures in the anterior and posterior lower leg. It is important to verify that the Hohmann retractors are positioned close to the bone; otherwise, the tendons and neurovascular structures are in danger of being injured. The osteotomy is performed using an oscillating

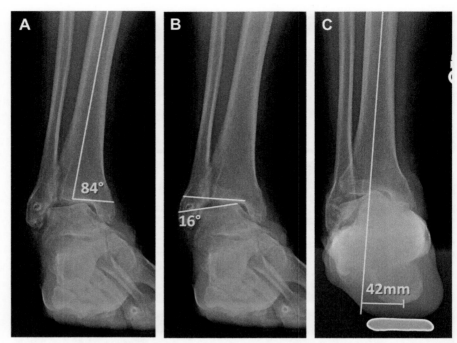

Fig. 5. Radiographic assessment of a varus deformity in the coronal plane (the same patient as in **Fig. 4**): (A) medial distal tibial angle; (B) tibiotalar tilt; (C) calcaneal moment arm.

saw while under permanent water irrigation to avoid or reduce heat damage, which may impair postoperative osseous healing. Because the contralateral cortex should remain preserved, fluoroscopy can inform when the osteotomy should be stopped before the lateral cortex is injured. The authors recommend using a chisel to carefully complete the osteotomy. After the osteotomy is performed, the authors use the K-wire–based distractor (eg, "Hintermann distractor") to open the osteotomy according to the preoperative plan. The osteotomy gap can be filled with an allograft (eg, femoral head/neck allograft) or an autograft (tricortical ipsilateral iliac crest bone graft). The osteotomy is stabilized using an anatomic T-shaped 3.5-mm plate. Despite all efforts to preserve the contralateral cortex, the cortex may be injured, especially in older patients because of their reduced bone elasticity. In that case, the authors recommend an additional lateral plate fixation through a separate incision (**Fig. 8**). After the osteotomy is fixed, the authors adapt the periosteum over the osteotomy with 2-0 absorbable sutures.

Supramalleolar Lateral Closing-Wedge Osteotomy

In patients with a preoperative varus deformity larger than 10° and/or a previously fused distal tibiofibular joint, a medial opening wedge osteotomy may not be feasible because of restriction through the fibula.[8,9,36,68] In these patients, a supramalleolar lateral closing-wedge osteotomy through the lateral approach is indicated. A Z-shaped osteotomy of the fibula is performed separately, using an oscillating saw to allow for adjustment of the final fibula length (**Fig. 9**). In patients with a fused distal tibiofibular joint, a lateral osteotomy can be performed en bloc (**Fig. 10**). For these

Table 2
Medial distal tibial angle for assessment of supramalleolar varus deformity

Normal Subjects	
Study	Mean MDTA
Chao et al,[50] 1994, radiographic study	92.9° ± 3.3°
Inman,[51] 1976, cadaver study	93.3° ± 3.2°
Knupp et al,[52] 2005, radiographic study	92.4° ± 3.1°
Paley et al,[53] 1994, radiographic study	91.4° ± 3.8°
Stufkens et al,[49] 2011, radiographic study	92.1° ± 2.2°

Patients with Varus Tibiotalar OA		
Study	Preoperative MDTA	Postoperative MDTA
Ahn et al,[31] 2015, 18 ankles	86.6° (85.7° to 87.6°)	92.9° (91.6° to 94.3°)
Cheng et al,[54] 2001, 18 ankles	81° (75° to 86°)	90° (89° to 93°)
Colin et al,[55] 2014, 62 ankles	76° ± 9°	91° ± 8°
Harstall et al,[33] 2007, 9 ankles	83.1° ± 3.8° (75° to 90°)	90.6° ± 1.9° (87° to 93°)
Hongmou et al,[34] 2016, 39 ankles	81.2° ± 3.0°	88.3° ± 2.5°
Jung et al,[56] 2017, 22 ankles	83.5°	93.8°
Kim et al,[35] 2014, 31 ankles	82.9° ± 2.1° (78.3° to 86.8°)	89.5° ± 1.9° (85.3° to 92.7°)
Kobayashi et al,[57] 2016, 27 ankles	84.9° (78° to 90°)	95.0° (83° to 99°)
Krähenbühl et al,[37] 2017, 99 ankles	85.1° ± 5.9°	91.4° ± 4.4°
Lee et al,[58] 2011, 16 ankles	84.7° ± 2.1°	99.6° ± 5.1°
Takakura et al,[59] 1995, 18 ankles	82.3°	93.8°
Takakura et al,[10] 1998, 9 ankles	70.0° ± 7.8° (54° to 78°)	87.1° ± 4.3° (78° to 92°)
Tanaka et al,[11] 2006, 26 ankles	82.7° (76° to 87°)	98.2° (90° to 113°)

Abbreviation: MDTA, medial distal tibial angle.

patients, the contralateral cortex should be preserved to ensure the initial stability of the osteotomy. A reversed K-wire–based distractor can be used to apply compression across the osteotomy. The authors recommend using plates for the final fixation of osteotomies.

Table 3
Tibiotalar tilt angle for assessment of intraarticular varus deformity

Patients with Varus Tibiotalar OA		
Study	Preoperative Tibiotalar Tilt	Postoperative Tibiotalar Tilt
Ahn et al,[31] 2015, 18 ankles	5.6° (4.8° to 6.6°)	5.5° (3.8° to 7.6°)
Colin et al,[55] 2014, 62 ankles	6° ± 8°	1° ± 3°
Hongmou et al,[34] 2016, 39 ankles	5.4° ± 4.1°	2.2° ± 1.7°
Jung et al,[56] 2017, 22 ankles	3.4°	2.2°
Kim et al,[35] 2014, 31 ankles	5.4° ± 1.4° (2.9° to 8.3°)	2.5° ± 1.8° (0.8° to 5.3°)
Kobayashi et al,[57] 2016, 27 ankles	8.3° ± 5.3°	1.8° ± 2.2°
Lee et al,[58] 2011, 16 ankles	6.6° ± 4.8°	4.5° ± 6.0°
Tanaka et al,[11] 2006, 26 ankles	7.3° (0° to 27°)	5.0° (-1° to 19°)

Table 4
Calcaneal moment measurement for assessment of inframalleolar varus deformity

	Patients with Varus Tibiotalar OA	
Study	Preoperative Calcaneal Moment	Postoperative Calcaneal Moment
Ahn et al,[31] 2015, 18 ankles	5.2° (3.1° to 7.2°)	2.1° (−0.5° to 4.6°)
Lee et al,[58] 2011, 16 ankles	−0.3° ± 10.6°	−8.2° ± 7.3°

Postoperative Rehabilitation

Postoperatively, the leg is placed in a lower-leg splint with plenty of cast padding. When wound conditions are appropriate, sutures can be removed 2 to 3 weeks after surgery. The authors then recommend transitioning to a lower-leg cast or a 3-dimensional tall walking boot with 10 kg. partial weight-bearing (able to touch the ground with the sole). The first clinical and radiographic follow-up is scheduled for 6 to 8 weeks postoperatively and includes non-weight-bearing radiographs. In patients with appropriate osseous healing, the authors recommend a gradual increase in weight-bearing, starting with 25% and further increasing by 25% every 3 to 5 days. After another 4 to 6 weeks, the authors recommend transitioning to normal shoes.

LITERATURE OVERVIEW: RESULTS AFTER SUPRAMALLEOLAR OSTEOTOMY

Currently, there are still a limited number of studies highlighting outcomes in patients who underwent SMOT (see **Table 5**).[30] SMOT remains a technically demanding procedure, and associated complications are not uncommon.[30]

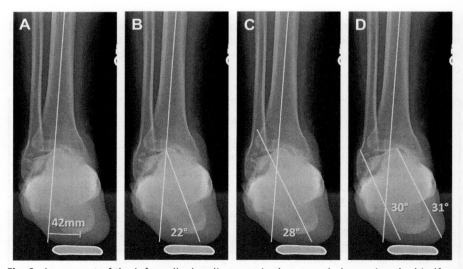

Fig. 6. Assessment of the inframalleolar alignment in the coronal plane using the hindfoot alignment view: (A) tuber calcanei distance; (B) tuber calcanei angle; (C) calcaneal/subtalar axis angle; (D) lateral and medial calcaneus contours angles.

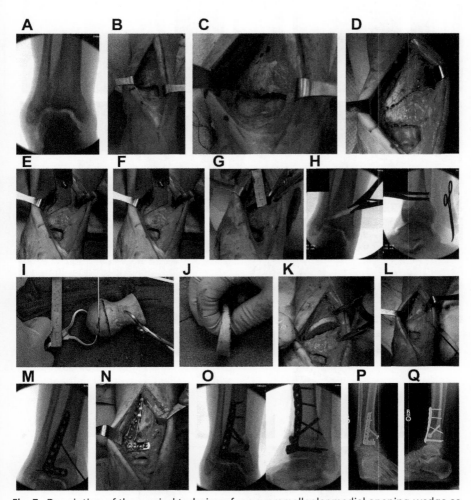

Fig. 7. Description of the surgical technique for a supramalleolar medial opening-wedge osteotomy (the same patient as in **Fig. 4**). (*A*) Valgus stress is applied to verify that varus talar tilt can be corrected. (*B*) A standard anterior approach exposes the tibiotalar joint. (*C*) Osteophytes on the tibial (especially anterolateral) and talar neck are removed. (*D*) The osteotomy line is marked according to preoperative planning. (*E*) The osteotomy is performed using an osteotome. (*F*) Several osteotomes with increasing thickness are used to mobilize the osteotomy. (*G*) A laminar spreader is used to preliminarily maintain the osteotomy gap. (*H*) Clinical and fluoroscopy checks are needed to ensure appropriate correction of the underlying deformity as well as appropriate alignment in both planes. (*I*) A femoral head is used to harvest (*J*) the tricortical structural allograft. (*K*) A K-wire–based spreader is used to mobilize the osteotomy for allograft insertion. (*L*) A K-wire is used for preliminary fixation of the allograft and the osteotomy, (*M*) which is checked using fluoroscopy. (*N*) Final fixation of the osteotomy using an anatomic plane and an axial screw. (*O*) A radiographic check demonstrates appropriate positioning of the hardware and good overall alignment. (*P*) Weight-bearing mortise and (*Q*) lateral views of the ankle at the 3-month follow-up demonstrate progressive healing of the osteotomy and neutral supramalleolar alignment.

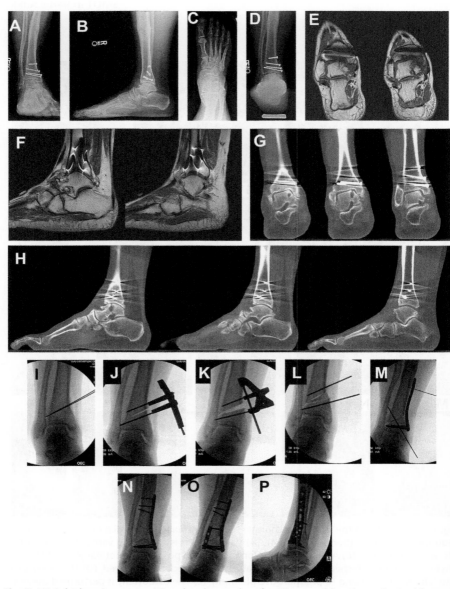

Fig. 8. Weight-bearing conventional radiographs of a 52-year-old male patient with post-traumatic tibiotalar OA. (*A*) Mortise view of the ankle. (*B*) Lateral and (*C*) dorsoplantar views of the foot. (*D*) Hindfoot alignment view. Medial distal tibial angle of 80°, a tibiotalar tilt of 12° varus, and a calcaneal moment arm of 27-mm varus. MRI, including (*E*) coronal T1 and (*F*) sagittal proton density (PD) weighted sequences, demonstrates asymmetric medial tibiotalar OA with cystic changes. WBCT scan, including (*G*) coronal and (*H*) sagittal slides, demonstrates medial tibiotalar OA with some incongruency of the joint space and varus talar tilt. (*I*) Intraoperative marking of the osteotomy plane using 2 parallel K-wires. (*J*) A K-wire–based spreader is used to open up the osteotomy (*K*) according to preoperative planning. (*L*) Femoral head tricortical allograft is used to fill up the osteotomy gap. (*M*) Preliminary transfixation of allograft and osteotomy using a K-wire. (*N*) Osteotomy fixation using a medial anatomic plate. (*O*) Additional fixation of the osteotomy using one-third tubular plate through the separate lateral incision. (*P*) Radiographic check demonstrates appropriate position of hardware and good overall alignment.

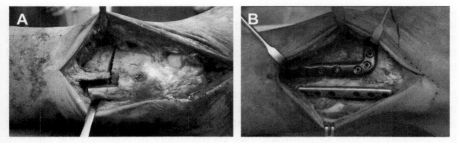

Fig. 9. (*A*) Lateral approach with a Z-shaped osteotomy of the fibula. (*B*) Plate fixation of the tibia and fibula.

Intraoperative complications include injury to the neurovascular structures and tendons in the anterior and posterior lower leg. Exact anatomic knowledge and protection of soft tissue by using Hohmann retractors are crucial to avoiding these injuries. When placing Hohmann retractors, the authors recommend ensuring that the retractors are

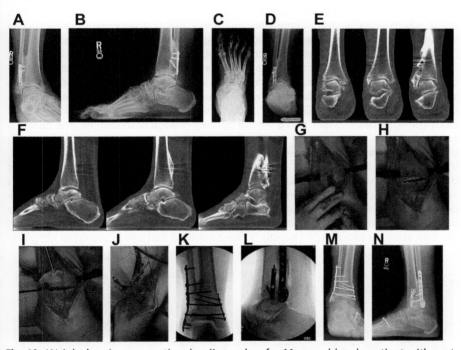

Fig. 10. Weight-bearing conventional radiographs of a 44-year-old male patient with post-traumatic tibiotalar OA. (*A*) Mortise view of the ankle. (*B*) Lateral and (*C*) dorsoplantar views of the foot. (*D*) Hindfoot alignment view. A medial distal tibial angle of 83°, a tibiotalar tilt of 11° varus, and a calcaneal moment arm of 32-mm varus. WBCT scan, including (*E*) coronal and (*F*) sagittal slides, demonstrates medial tibiotalar OA with some incongruency of the joint space, varus talar tilt, and osseous fusion of the distal tibiofibular syndesmosis. (*G*, *H*) Lateral osteotomy is performed en bloc. (*I*) Lateral osseous wedge is removed. (*J*) A K-wire reversed distractor is used to apply compression across the osteotomy site. (*K* and *L*) Final fixation of both osteotomies using 2 plates. (*M*) Weight-bearing mortise and (*N*) lateral views of the ankle at the 3-month follow-up demonstrate progressive healing of both osteotomies and neutral supramalleolar alignment.

placed close to the tibia and not external to the tendons (**Fig. 11**). As mentioned before, mobilizing the osteotomy (closing or opening) may result in accidental injury of the contralateral cortex. Therefore, the authors recommend additional fixation of the osteotomy through a separate incision before distraction if there is suspicion of lateral cortical issues (see **Fig. 8**).

Perioperative complications include thromboembolic complications. Wound-healing problems, including deep infection, have an incidence of up to 22% in the current literature.[30] Early superficial infection can be treated by antibiotic application. However, in patients with deep infection, surgical debridement and possibly removal of hardware may be necessary to eradicate the infection (**Fig. 12**).

Delayed union or nonunion is a possible major postoperative complication of SMOT. In the available literature, the incidence of this type of complication can be as high as 22%.[30] Factors specific to surgical technique may play an important role in explaining delayed union or nonunion: injury of the contralateral cortex, anatomic repositioning, appropriate fixation of the osteotomy, opening- versus closing-wedge osteotomy, and the use of autograft versus allograft to fill the osteotomy gap in patients with an opening-wedge osteotomy. In the authors' previous study, which included 16 patients who underwent SMOT, they compared outcomes in patients with opening-wedge versus closing-wedge osteotomy.[32] The time until complete osseous union was significantly shorter in patients with closing-wedge SMOT (2.3 ± 0.4 months vs 5.4 ± 5.5 months, P = .008). Two patients with opening-wedge osteotomies had delayed osseous union, whereas all patients with closing-wedge osteotomies united within 6 months.[32] Similar results were observed in a study by Stamatis and colleagues,[69] which included 7 medial closing-wedge osteotomies and 6 medial opening-wedge osteotomies. The osseous unions occurred at a mean of 10.6 ± 5.2 and 18.2 ± 9.8 weeks in patients with closing-wedge and opening-wedge SMOT, respectively.[69] In the current literature, there is no evidence whether autografts or allografts have a lower incidence of delayed union or nonunion. Interestingly, in a previous study, the authors analyzed secondary loss of hindfoot alignment and graft incorporation in 50 patients who underwent lateral lengthening osteotomies of the calcaneus.[70] Twenty-five of these patients underwent an autologous iliac crest autograft, whereas 25 patients underwent an acellular allograft.[70] This study demonstrated that use of sterilized allografts

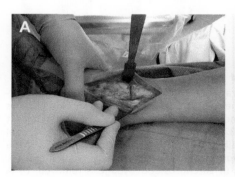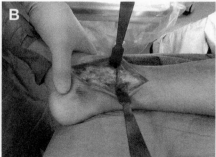

Fig. 11. Medial distal tibial approach for medial opening wedge osteotomy in a 24-year-old female patient. (*A*) Close relationship of posterior tibial tendon to posterior periosteum of the tibia. (*B*) Both Hohmann hooks are placed close to the tibia to ensure that tendons and neurovascular structures are protected.

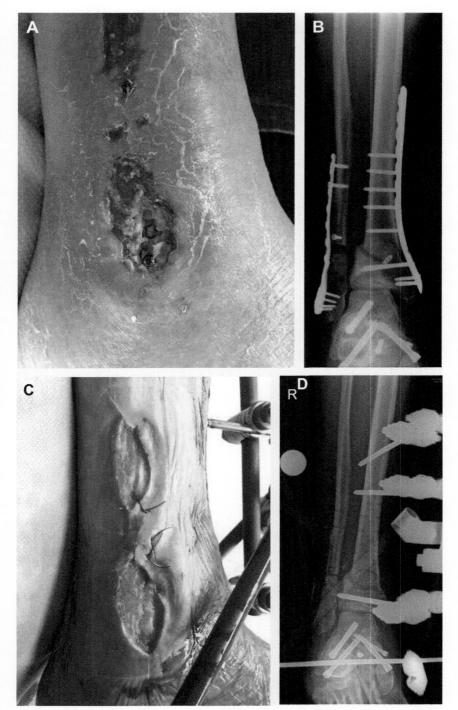

Fig. 12. (*A*, *B*) Deep infection with skin defect exposing hardware on the lateral side 6 weeks status post reconstructive surgery. (*C*, *D*) Deep debridement, removal of hardware, and application of external fixator were performed. Secondary wound healing was initiated.

Table 5
Complications and functional outcomes in patients who underwent supramalleolar osteotomy for varus deformity

Study	Study Type	Patients with Varus OA	Surgical Technique	Follow-up (y)	Complications			Functional Outcome
					Intraoperative	Perioperative	Postoperative	
Ahn et al,[31] 2015	RS, SC	18	MOW OT (18)	2.8 (2–5.5)	Intraarticular cartilage damage by OT (1)	None	• Painful hardware (9) with ROH (7) • Progression of ankle OA requiring TAR (1)	• VAS: 6.7 → 2.7 • AOFAS: 78.4 → 89
Cheng et al,[54] 2001	RS, SC	18	MOW OT with fibula OT (18)	4.0 (2.1–6.8)	None	Late infection requiring ROH (1)	• Delayed union with implant failure requiring revision (2)	Pain: 24.4 → 47.5
Colin et al,[55] 2014	RS, SC	62	LCW (41) or MOW (21) OT	3.5 (1–14)	None	Delayed wound healing (1)	• Overcorrection requiring revision (1) • Impingement requiring debridement (1) • Nonunion requiring revision (1) • Progression of ankle OA requiring ankle AD (1)	AOFAS: 58 → 73
Harstall et al,[33] 2007	RS, SC	9	LCW OT with fibula OT (9)	4.7 (1.3–7.3)	None	None	• ROH (2) • Progression of OA (2) requiring ankle AD (1)	AOFAS: 48 (21–67) → 74 (51–88) AOFAS pain: 16 (0–20) → 30 (20–40)
Hintermann et al,[72] 2017	PS, SC	20	Intraarticular MOW OT (20)	5.9 (4–11.2)	None	None	• ROH (5)	• VAS: 7.9 ± 1.3 → 1.3 ± 1.6 • AOFAS: 49 ± 15 → 86 ± 12

Study	Design, n	Procedure (n)	Follow-up (y)				Outcomes
Hongmou et al,[34] 2016	RS, SC 39	MOW OT with (21) or without (18) fibula OT	3.1 (1.4–5.1)	None	None	• Delayed union (3) • Progression of ankle OA requiring ankle AD (2)	• AOFAS: 51 ± 14 → 83 ± 10 • Maryland: 58 ± 12 → 82 ± 6 • AOS pain: 43 ± 5.5 → 26 ± 5 • AOS function: 53 ± 12 → 37 ± 10.5
Jung et al,[56] 2017	RS, SC 22	MOW OT with fibula OT (22)	2.0 (1–5)	None	None	• Delayed union (1) • Malunion (1)	• VAS: 6.5 → 1.1 • AOFAS: 61 → 87
Kim et al,[35] 2014	RS, SC 31	MOW OT (31)	2.3 (2–2.8)	n.r.	n.r.	Progression of OA (13)	VAS: 7.1 ± 0.8 → 4.1 ± 1.6 AOFAS: 63 ± 4 → 80 ± 8
Knupp et al,[36] 2008	RS, SC 12	LCW or MOW OT with fibula OT (12)	5 (3–10.5)	n.r.	n.r.	n.r.	VAS: 7 (4–10) → 3 (1–6)
Knupp et al,[20] 2012	RS, SC 29	LCW (12) or MOW (17) OT	3.8	n.r.	n.r.	• ROH (9) • Progression of ankle OA requiring TAR (1)	• VAS: 4.4 → 2.6 • AOFAS: 52 → 73
Kobayashi et al,[57] 2016	RS, SC 27	MOW OT (27)	2.3 (1.2–3.8)	Unstable lateral hinge fracture (1)	• Hematoma (2) • Superficial infection (1) • Tarsal tunnel syndrome (1)	• Secondary loss of correction after early ROH (1)	• VAS: 7.4 ± 3.1 → 2.1 ± 1.6 • AOFAS: 59 ± 16 → 89 ± 12 • Takakura score: 56 ± 16 → 85 ± 17
Krähenbühl et al,[37] 2017	PS, SC 99	LCW or MOW OT with (33) or without (66) fibula OT	5.0 ± 3.7	n.r.	n.r.	• Deep infection (2) • Nonunion (3) • Re-OT (4) • Progression of ankle OA requiring ankle AD (3) or TAR (14) • ROH (56)	• VAS: 4.5 ± 1.7 → 3.0 ± 2.3 • AOFAS: 53 ± 17 → 73 ± 18

(continued on next page)

Table 5
(continued)

Study	Study Type	Patients with Varus OA	Surgical Technique	Follow-up (y)	Intraoperative	Perioperative	Postoperative	Functional Outcome
					Complications			
Lee et al,[58] 2011	PS, SC	16	MOW OT with fibula OT (16)	2.3 (1–6.5)	n.r.	n.r.	n.r.	AOFAS: 62 ± 9 → 82 ± 11
Mann et al,[73] 2012	RS, SC	19	Intraarticular MOW OT (19)	4.9 (1.2–8.2)	n.r.	n.r.	Progression of ankle OA requiring TAR (2)	AOFAS: 46 → 78
Takakura et al,[59] 1995	PS, SC	18	MOW OT (18)	6.8 (2.6–12.8)	n.r.	n.r.	• Delayed union (1)	• Pain: 16.4 → 34.6 • Walking ability: 11.7 → 16.7 • Activities of daily living: 12.5 → 16.5
Takakura et al,[10] 1998	PS, SC	9	MOW OT (9)	7.3 (2.3–13.2)	n.r.	n.r.	• Decrease of ROM (6) • Persisting pain (4)	• Takakura score: 68.9 → 87.2 • Pain: 20 → 34.4 • Walking ability: 15.6 → 18.9 • Activities of daily living: 14.7 → 16.9
Tanaka et al,[11] 2006	RS, SC	26	MOW OT with fibula OT (26)	8.3 (2.3–17.9)	n.r.	n.r.	• Nonunion requiring bone grafting (4) • ROH (18) • Progression of OA (4) requiring ankle AD (2)	• Takakura score: 51 → 79 • Pain: 14.2 → 33.1

Abbreviations: AD, arthrodesis; AOFAS, American Orthopaedic Foot and Ankle Society; AOS, ankle osteoarthritis scale; LCW, lateral closing wedge; MOW, medial opening wedge; n.r., not reported; OA, osteoarthritis; OT, osteotomy; PS, prospective; ROH, removal of hardware; ROM, range of motion; RS, retrospective; SC, single center; TAR, total ankle replacement; VAS, visual analog scale; y, years.

does not increase the incidence of complications, including secondary loss of correction and nonunion.[70]

Although SMOT may slow the progression of tibiotalar degeneration, up to 25% of all patients who underwent SMOT have substantial progression of OA at midterm follow-up, requiring ankle arthrodesis or total ankle replacement.[30] In a prospective study by Krähenbühl and colleagues[37] with 99 varus osteoarthritic ankles, 17 patients underwent secondary procedures, including 14 total ankle replacements (mean time 3.2 years after the index surgery with a range between 0.6 and 12.7 years) and 3 ankle arthrodeses (mean time 5.1 years after the index surgery with a range between 0.6 and 13 years).[37] Kim and colleagues[35] retrospectively evaluated 31 ankles that underwent a medial opening-wedge SMOT. In all patients, arthroscopic bone marrow stimulation was performed on medial cartilage lesions. In all patients, the second-look arthroscopy and removal of hardware were performed at a mean of 13.2 ± 1.4 months after the index surgery. At that time, most patients reported significant pain relief (visual analog scale [VAS] 7.1 ± 0.8 → 3.4 ± 1.3) and functional improvement (American Orthopedic Foot and Ankle Society [AOFAS] hindfoot score 62.9 ± 4.0 → 83.1 ± 7.5). At the second-look arthroscopy, cartilage degeneration was evaluated using the International Cartilage Repair Society grade and was classified as normal in 1 (3%), nearly normal in 7 (23%), abnormal in 13 (42%), and severely abnormal in 10 (32%) ankles. Progressive degeneration of the tibiotalar joint was observed in 13 patients (42%). At the final follow-up approximately 1 year after the second-look arthroscopy, both VAS and AOFAS substantially worsened.[35] One possible reason SMOT failure requires a joint-sacrificing procedure is the omission of osteochondral lesions as a contraindication for SMOT. Active bipolar osteochondral lesions have been demonstrated to be a risk factor for poor outcomes in patients who underwent SMOT.[71]

Promising short- and midterm results have been reported in the available literature (**Table 5**).[30] However, *complete pain relief should not be expected following a SMOT procedure* (see **Table 5**). Although the surgery may result in perfect restoration of hindfoot alignment, preexisting degenerative changes of the tibiotalar joint are often irreversible, as mentioned above. Another possible explanation for remaining ankle pain is that SMOT is a powerful tool for correction of supramalleolar deformity in the coronal plane (as assessed using medial distal tibial angle), but the intraarticular deformity (as assessed by tibiotalar tilt) may be reduced but not completely corrected (see **Table 3**). The authors' experience is that, on average, the varus tibiotalar tilt can be reduced by half (**Fig. 13**),[32] which is similar to other reports.[34] A preoperative varus tibiotalar tilt of more than 7° has been demonstrated to be a potential predictor for worse postoperative results.[22,31,58] Ahn and colleagues[31] performed medial opening-wedge osteotomies without fibular osteotomy on 18 patients who were followed for between 2 and 5.5 years. The mean medial distal tibial angle improved significantly from 86.6° (95% confidence interval [CI]: 85.7° to 87.6°) to 92.2° (95% CI: 91.6° to 94.3°). However, the mean talar tilt angle remained the same preoperatively 5.6° (95% CI: 4.8° to 6.6°) as postoperatively 5.5° (95% CI: 3.8° to 7.6°) ($P = .916$). In total, talar tilt increased by less than 2° in 4 ankles and decreased by greater than 2° in 3 ankles. The investigators explained this less than favorable outcome by the fact that SMOT is an extraarticular procedure that does not change the shape of the ankle mortise.[31] Another reason for persisting varus talar tilt is that SMOT may be insufficient to reorient the talus because of asymmetric joint wear.[72] A possible approach to address this problem is the intraarticular distal tibia osteotomy (so-called plafondplasty).[13,15,23,73] Hintermann and colleagues[72] modified this surgical technique by adding a medial opening wedge osteotomy to plafondplasty (**Fig. 14**).

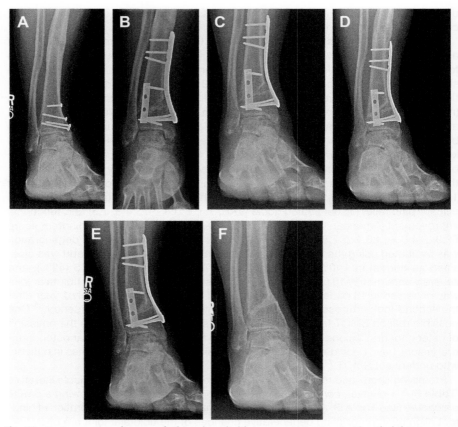

Fig. 13. Postoperative change of tibiotalar tilt (the same patient as in **Fig. 8**). (*A*) Preoperative weight-bearing mortise view of the ankle demonstrates tibiotalar tilt of 12° varus. (*B*) Postoperative non-weight-bearing mortise view of the ankle demonstrates tibiotalar tilt of 9°. Postoperative weight-bearing mortise view of the ankle demonstrates tibiotalar tilt (*C*) of 9° at 3 months, (*D*) 8° at 6 months, (*E*) 8° at 12 months, and (*F*) 9° at 15 months (3 months after removal of hardware).

Favorable outcomes, including pain relief and functional improvement, were demonstrated at the mean follow-up of 5.9 years with a range between 4 and 11.2 years. The talar tilt improved significantly from 19.4° ± 8.2° (range 6° to 32°) to 6.9° ± 3.9° (range 1° to 12°). No midterm complications, including progression of tibiotalar OA, were observed in this study.[72] However, further long-term studies are needed to confirm these favorable results. One of the critical technical points of this procedure is the intraarticular course of osteotomy with inevitable damage of joint cartilage on the tibial side. Tochigi and colleagues[74] performed a cadaver study with 7 normal human ankles harvested immediately following amputation. Transarticular compressive impaction was applied to mimic the intraarticular tibial plafond fracture. Chondrocyte viability was analyzed, and chondrocyte death was demonstrated to be significantly higher in fracture-edge regions. Furthermore, progression of cell death was observed over the next 48 hours with 25.9% of fractional cell death along fracture lines versus 8.6% in nonfracture regions.[74]

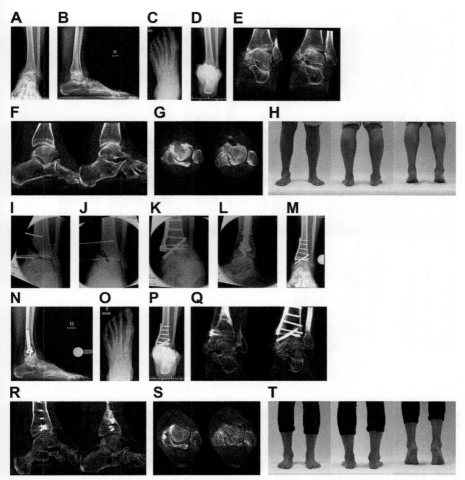

Fig. 14. Weight-bearing conventional radiographs of a 46-year-old female patient with post-traumatic ligamentous tibiotalar OA. (*A*) Mortise view of the ankle. (*B*) Lateral and (*C*) dorso-plantar views of the foot. (*D*) Hindfoot alignment view. WBCT scan, including (*E*) coronal, (*F*) sagittal, and (*G*) axial slides, demonstrates varus tibiotalar OA with partially preserved lateral compartment, severe varus tilt, and incongruency of the tibiotalar joint. (*H*) Clinical assessment demonstrates varus alignment of the right hindfoot. (*I*) First, intraarticular plafondplasty was performed. (*J*) An allograft was used to fill up the osteotomy. (*K, L*) Second, an additional medial opening wedge SMOT of the distal tibia was performed. Weight-bearing conventional radiographs at the 3-year follow-up. (*M*) Mortise view of the ankle. (*N*) Lateral and (*O*) dorso-plantar views of the foot. (*P*) Hindfoot alignment view. WBCT scan at a 3-year follow-up, including (*Q*) coronal, (*R*) sagittal, and (*S*) axial slides, demonstrates improved hindfoot alignment. (*T*) Clinical assessment demonstrates neutral alignment of the right hindfoot. (*Courtesy of* Professor Beat Hintermann, MD, Kantonsspital Baselland, Liestal, Switzerland.)

SUMMARY

SMOT often results in promising short- and midterm results as reported in the current literature.[30] As simple as it sounds, the primary indication for SMOT is a deformity at the *supramalleolar* and not at the *inframalleolar* level (**Fig. 15**). SMOT is a reliable

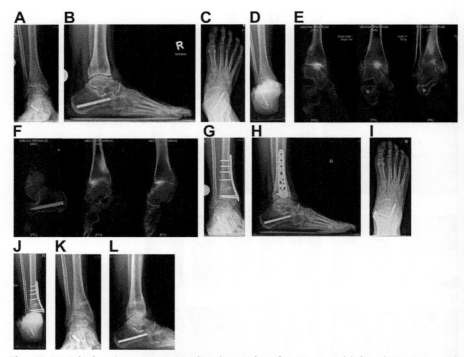

Fig. 15. Weight-bearing conventional radiographs of a 24-year-old female patient with posttraumatic tibiotalar OA. (*A*) Mortise view of the ankle. (*B*) Lateral and (*C*) dorsoplantar views of the foot. (*D*) Hindfoot alignment view. One year ago, patient underwent a lateral lengthening osteotomy of the calcaneus without any success. Single-photon emission computed tomography-CT scan, including (*E*) coronal and (*F*) sagittal slides, demonstrates degeneration of the medial tibiotalar joint with enhancement. Weight-bearing conventional radiographs at 9-month follow-up after a supramalleolar medial opening-wedge osteotomy. (*G*) Mortise view of the ankle. (*H*) Lateral and (*I*) dorsoplantar views of the foot. (*J*) Hindfoot alignment view. (*K*) Mortise view and (*L*) lateral view after removal of hardware (12 months after the index procedure).

treatment option in patients with asymmetric ankle degeneration and concomitant *supramalleolar* varus deformity. However, the complications associated with this procedure are not uncommon. Complete degeneration of the tibiotalar joint can occur in up to 25% of all patients within 10 years, requiring another major procedure like ankle arthrodesis or total ankle replacement, and thus, patients should be thoroughly informed of this possibility. Further long-term studies are needed to identify the risk factors for failure of this procedure and to improve patient care.

REFERENCES

1. Saltzman CL, Salamon ML, Blanchard GM, et al. Epidemiology of ankle arthritis: report of a consecutive series·of 639 patients from a tertiary orthopaedic center. Iowa Orthop J 2005;25(1):44–6.
2. Valderrabano V, Horisberger M, Russell I, et al. Etiology of ankle osteoarthritis. Clin Orthop Relat Res 2009;467(7):1800–6.
3. Horisberger M, Valderrabano V, Hintermann B. Posttraumatic ankle osteoarthritis after ankle-related fractures. J Orthop Trauma 2009;23(1):60–7.

4. Lubbeke A, Salvo D, Stern R, et al. Risk factors for post-traumatic osteoarthritis of the ankle: an eighteen year follow-up study. Int Orthop 2012;36(7):1403–10.
5. Valderrabano V, Hintermann B, Horisberger M, et al. Ligamentous posttraumatic ankle osteoarthritis. Am J Sports Med 2006;34(4):612–20.
6. Barg A, Pagenstert GI, Hugle T, et al. Ankle osteoarthritis: etiology, diagnostics, and classification. Foot Ankle Clin 2013;18(3):411–26.
7. Wang B, Saltzman CL, Chalayon O, et al. Does the subtalar joint compensate for ankle malalignment in end-stage ankle arthritis? Clin Orthop Relat Res 2015; 473(1):318–25.
8. Knupp M, Stufkens SA, Bolliger L, et al. Classification and treatment of supramalleolar deformities. Foot Ankle Int 2011;32(11):1023–31.
9. Stufkens SA, Van Bergen CJ, Blankevoort L, et al. The role of the fibula in varus and valgus deformity of the tibia: a biomechanical study. J Bone Joint Surg Br 2011;93(9):1232–9.
10. Takakura Y, Takaoka T, Tanaka Y, et al. Results of opening-wedge osteotomy for the treatment of a post-traumatic varus deformity of the ankle. J Bone Joint Surg Am 1998;80(2):213–8.
11. Tanaka Y, Takakura Y, Hayashi K, et al. Low tibial osteotomy for varus-type osteoarthritis of the ankle. J Bone Joint Surg Br 2006;88(7):909–13.
12. Speed JS, Boyd HB. Operative reconstruction of malunited fractures about the ankle joint. J Bone Joint Surg Am 1936;18(2):270–86.
13. Al-Nammari SS, Myerson MS. The use of tibial osteotomy (ankle plafondplasty) for joint preservation of ankle deformity and early arthritis. Foot Ankle Clin 2016;21(1):15–26.
14. Barg A, Pagenstert GI, Horisberger M, et al. Supramalleolar osteotomies for degenerative joint disease of the ankle joint: indication, technique and results. Int Orthop 2013;37(9):1683–95.
15. Becker AS, Myerson MS. The indications and technique of supramalleolar osteotomy. Foot Ankle Clin 2009;14(3):549–61.
16. Benthien RA, Myerson MS. Supramalleolar osteotomy for ankle deformity and arthritis. Foot Ankle Clin 2004;9(3):475–87.
17. Easley ME. Surgical treatment of the arthritic varus ankle. Foot Ankle Clin 2012; 17(4):665–86.
18. Hintermann B, Knupp M, Barg A. Supramalleolar osteotomies for the treatment of ankle arthritis. J Am Acad Orthop Surg 2016;24(7):424–32.
19. Knupp M. The use of osteotomies in the treatment of asymmetric ankle joint arthritis. Foot Ankle Int 2017;38(2):220–9.
20. Knupp M, Bolliger L, Hintermann B. Treatment of posttraumatic varus ankle deformity with supramalleolar osteotomy. Foot Ankle Clin 2012;17(1):95–102.
21. Krause F, Veljkovic A, Schmid T. Supramalleolar osteotomies for posttraumatic malalignment of the distal tibia. Foot Ankle Clin 2016;21(1):1–14.
22. Lee WC. Extraarticular supramalleolar osteotomy for managing varus ankle osteoarthritis, alternatives for osteotomy: how and why? Foot Ankle Clin 2016;21(1): 27–35.
23. Myerson MS, Zide JR. Management of varus ankle osteoarthritis with joint-preserving osteotomy. Foot Ankle Clin 2013;18(3):471–80.
24. Stamatis ED, Myerson MS. Supramalleolar osteotomy: indications and technique. Foot Ankle Clin 2003;8(2):317–33.
25. Tanaka Y. The concept of ankle joint preserving surgery: why does supramalleolar osteotomy work and how to decide when to do an osteotomy or joint replacement. Foot Ankle Clin 2012;17(4):545–53.

26. Barg A, Elsner A, Anderson AE, et al. The effect of three-component total ankle replacement malalignment on clinical outcome: pain relief and functional outcome in 317 consecutive patients. J Bone Joint Surg Am 2011;93(21): 1969–78.

27. Cenni F, Leardini A, Cheli A, et al. Position of the prosthesis components in total ankle replacement and the effect on motion at the replaced joint. Int Orthop 2012; 36(3):571–8.

28. Espinosa N, Walti M, Favre P, et al. Misalignment of total ankle components can induce high joint contact pressures. J Bone Joint Surg Am 2010;92(5):1179–87.

29. Tochigi Y, Rudert MJ, Brown TD, et al. The effect of accuracy of implantation on range of movement of the Scandinavian Total Ankle Replacement. J Bone Joint Surg Br 2005;87(5):736–40.

30. Barg A, Saltzman CL. Single-stage supramalleolar osteotomy for coronal plane deformity. Curr Rev Musculoskelet Med 2014;7(4):277–91.

31. Ahn TK, Yi Y, Cho JH, et al. A cohort study of patients undergoing distal tibial osteotomy without fibular osteotomy for medial ankle arthritis with mortise widening. J Bone Joint Surg Am 2015;97(5):381–8.

32. Barg A, Wiewiorski M, Paul J, et al. Supramalleolar osteotomy in asymmetric ankle osteoarthritis: short-term clinical and radiographic results. Orthopade 2017;46(9):761–75 [in German].

33. Harstall R, Lehmann O, Krause F, et al. Supramalleolar lateral closing wedge osteotomy for the treatment of varus ankle arthrosis. Foot Ankle Int 2007;28(5): 542–8.

34. Hongmou Z, Xiaojun L, Yi L, et al. Supramalleolar osteotomy with or without fibular osteotomy for varus ankle arthritis. Foot Ankle Int 2016;37(9):1001–7.

35. Kim YS, Park EH, Koh YG, et al. Supramalleolar osteotomy with bone marrow stimulation for varus ankle osteoarthritis: clinical results and second-look arthroscopic evaluation. Am J Sports Med 2014;42(7):1558–66.

36. Knupp M, Pagenstert G, Valderrabano V, et al. Osteotomies in varus malalignment of the ankle. Oper Orthop Traumatol 2008;20(3):262–73 [in German].

37. Krähenbühl N, Zwicky L, Bolliger L, et al. Mid- to long-term results of supramalleolar osteotomy. Foot Ankle Int 2017;38(2):124–32.

38. Gortler H, Rusyn J, Godbout C, et al. Diabetes and healing outcomes in lower extremity fractures: a systematic review. Injury 2018;49(2):177–83.

39. Marin C, Luyten FP, Van Der Schueren B, et al. The impact of type 2 diabetes on bone fracture healing. Front Endocrinol (Lausanne) 2018;9:6.

40. Lee JJ, Patel R, Biermann JS, et al. The musculoskeletal effects of cigarette smoking. J Bone Joint Surg Am 2013;95(9):850–9.

41. Barg A. Conventional imaging of the hindfoot and Saltzman view. Fuss Sprungg 2015;13(2):58–77. [in German].

42. Saltzman CL, El-Khoury GY. The hindfoot alignment view. Foot Ankle Int 1995; 16(9):572–6.

43. Norton AA, Callaghan JJ, Amendola A, et al. Correlation of knee and hindfoot deformities in advanced knee OA: compensatory hindfoot alignment and where it occurs. Clin Orthop Relat Res 2015;473(1):166–74.

44. Haraguchi N, Ota K, Tsunoda N, et al. Weight-bearing-line analysis in supramalleolar osteotomy for varus-type osteoarthritis of the ankle. J Bone Joint Surg Am 2015;97(4):333–9.

45. Paley D. Principles of deformity correction. Berlin: Springer; 2002.

46. Barg A, Bailey T, Richter M, et al. Weightbearing computed tomography of the foot and ankle: emerging technology topical review. Foot Ankle Int 2018;39(3): 376–86.
47. Barg A, Harris MD, Henninger HB, et al. Medial distal tibial angle: comparison between weightbearing mortise view and hindfoot alignment view. Foot Ankle Int 2012;33(8):655–61.
48. Barg A, Amendola RL, Henninger HB, et al. Measurement of supramalleolar alignment on the anteroposterior and hindfoot alignment views: influence of ankle position and radiographic projection angle. Foot Ankle Int 2015;36(11):1352–61.
49. Stufkens SA, Barg A, Bolliger L, et al. Measurement of the medial distal tibial angle. Foot Ankle Int 2011;32(3):288–93.
50. Chao EY, Neluheni EV, Hsu RW, et al. Biomechanics of malalignment. Orthop Clin North Am 1994;25(3):379–86.
51. Inman VT. The joints of the ankle. Baltimore (MD): Williams & Wilkins; 1976.
52. Knupp M, Ledermann H, Magerkurth O, et al. The surgical tibiotalar angle: a radiologic study. Foot Ankle Int 2005;26(9):713–6.
53. Paley D, Herzenberg JE, Tetsworth K, et al. Deformity planning for frontal and sagittal plane corrective osteotomies. Orthop Clin North Am 1994;25(3):425–65.
54. Cheng YM, Huang PJ, Hong SH, et al. Low tibial osteotomy for moderate ankle arthritis. Arch Orthop Trauma Surg 2001;121(6):355–8.
55. Colin F, Gaudot F, Odri G, et al. Supramalleolar osteotomy: techniques, indications and outcomes in a series of 83 cases. Orthop Traumatol Surg Res 2014; 100(4):413–8.
56. Jung HG, Lee DO, Lee SH, et al. Second-look arthroscopic evaluation and clinical outcome after supramalleolar osteotomy for medial compartment ankle osteoarthritis. Foot Ankle Int 2017;38(12):1311–7.
57. Kobayashi H, Kageyama Y, Shido Y. Treatment of varus ankle osteoarthritis and instability with a novel mortise-plasty osteotomy procedure. J Foot Ankle Surg 2016;55(1):60–7.
58. Lee WC, Moon JS, Lee K, et al. Indications for supramalleolar osteotomy in patients with ankle osteoarthritis and varus deformity. J Bone Joint Surg Am 2011; 93(13):1243–8.
59. Takakura Y, Tanaka Y, Kumai T, et al. Low tibial osteotomy for osteoarthritis of the ankle. Results of a new operation in 18 patients. J Bone Joint Surg Br 1995;77(1): 50–4.
60. Cox JS, Hewes TF. "Normal" talar tilt angle. Clin Orthop Relat Res 1979;140(1): 37–41.
61. Cobey JC. Posterior roentgenogram of the foot. Clin Orthop Relat Res 1976;118: 202–7.
62. Donovan A, Rosenberg ZS. Extraarticular lateral hindfoot impingement with posterior tibial tendon tear: MRI correlation. AJR Am J Roentgenol 2009;193(3): 672–8.
63. Knupp M, Stufkens SA, Pagenstert GI, et al. Supramalleolar osteotomy for tibiotalar varus malalignment. Tech Foot & Ankle 2009;8(1):17–23.
64. Warnock KM, Johnson BD, Wright JB, et al. Calculation of the opening wedge for a low tibial osteotomy. Foot Ankle Int 2004;25(11):778–82.
65. Golano P, Vega J, Perez-Carro L, et al. Ankle anatomy for the arthroscopist. Part II: role of the ankle ligaments in soft tissue impingement. Foot Ankle Clin 2006; 11(2):275–96.
66. Golano P, Vega J, Perez-Carro L, et al. Ankle anatomy for the arthroscopist. Part I: the portals. Foot Ankle Clin 2006;11(2):253–73.

67. Outerbridge RE. The etiology of chondromalacia patellae. J Bone Joint Surg Br 1961;43-b:752–7.
68. Knupp M, Stufkens SA, Van Bergen CJ, et al. Effect of supramalleolar varus and valgus deformities on the tibiotalar joint: a cadaveric study. Foot Ankle Int 2011; 32(6):609–15.
69. Stamatis ED, Cooper PS, Myerson MS. Supramalleolar osteotomy for the treatment of distal tibial angular deformities and arthritis of the ankle joint. Foot Ankle Int 2003;24(10):754–64.
70. Muller SA, Barg A, Vavken P, et al. Autograft versus sterilized allograft for lateral calcaneal lengthening osteotomies: comparison of 50 patients. Medicine (Baltimore) 2016;95(30):e4343.
71. Gross CE, Barfield W, Schweizer C, et al. The utility of the ankle SPECT/CT scan to predict functional and clinical outcomes in supramalleolar osteotomy patients. J Orthop Res 2018;36(7):2015–21.
72. Hintermann B, Ruiz R, Barg A. Novel double osteotomy technique of distal tibia for correction of asymmetric varus osteoarthritic ankle. Foot Ankle Int 2017; 38(9):970–81.
73. Mann HA, Filippi J, Myerson MS. Intra-articular opening medial tibial wedge osteotomy (plafond-plasty) for the treatment of intra-articular varus ankle arthritis and instability. Foot Ankle Int 2012;33(4):255–61.
74. Tochigi Y, Buckwalter JA, Martin JA, et al. Distribution and progression of chondrocyte damage in a whole-organ model of human ankle intra-articular fracture. J Bone Joint Surg Am 2011;93(6):533–9.

Arthrodesis of a Varus Ankle

Faisal AlSayel, MD[a], Victor Valderrabano, MD, PhD[b],*

KEYWORDS

- Varus ankle • Ankle arthrodesis • Ankle fusion • Ankle osteoarthritis • Cavovarus

KEY POINTS

- Corrective ankle arthrodesis for varus ankle osteoarthritis or severe cavovarus deformities is a challenging operation.
- To have a satisfactory outcome, concomitant procedures are often required.
- The main goal of surgery is to create a pain-free, stable, plantigrade foot.
- Different surgical approaches and techniques have been described in the literature.

INTRODUCTION

Varus ankle osteoarthritis (OA) with or without pes cavovarus is a challenging condition to treat. It typically results in pain, stiffness, dysfunction, and impaired mobility for the patient. There is normally loss of cartilage on the medial talar dome and/or medial gutter of the tibiotalar joint. It is characterized by malpositioning of the talus including medial translation of the talus, internal rotation along the longitudinal talus axis, and/or varus talar tilt.[1] Under weight-bearing, the malpositioning of the talus induces an eccentric load on the ankle, which can worsen the varus cartilage degeneration.

Valderrabano and colleagues[2] have shown that the average tibiotalar alignment is varus regardless of the underlying cause in most patients with ankle OA. It has been found by several authors that the varus alignment may be one component of a multiplanar deformity and is often associated with concomitant sagittal plane malposition on the lateral radiograph.[3–5] With recent advances in imaging, weight-bearing computed tomography has shown that varus ankle OA is a coronal plane and an axial plane deformity.[6] There is an increased incidence of abnormal internal rotation of the talus when compared with a normal control group, which occurred more frequently in severe varus ankle OA.

Before consideration of surgical intervention, conservative treatment, such as custom-made orthotics, ankle braces, walkers, and analgesic medications need to

Disclosure: The authors have nothing to disclose.
[a] Swiss Ortho Center, Schmerzklinik Basel, Swiss Medical Network, Hirschgässlein 15, 4010 Basel, Switzerland; [b] Swiss Ortho Center, University of Basel, Schmerzklinik Basel, Swiss Medical Network, Hirschgässlein 15, 4010 Basel, Switzerland
* Corresponding author.
E-mail address: vvalderrabano@swissmedical.net

Foot Ankle Clin N Am 24 (2019) 265–280
https://doi.org/10.1016/j.fcl.2019.02.009
foot.theclinics.com

be used first.[7] Varus ankle OA exists as a continuum. Therefore, the treating surgeon needs to be familiar with the various surgical options, which include joint-sparing ankle realignment, ankle arthrodesis, and total ankle arthroplasty with additional cosurgeries. Corrective ankle arthrodesis remains the most commonly used technique in the treatment of end-stage varus ankle OA. The main goal of surgery is to create a pain-free, stable, plantigrade hindfoot and foot.

The scope of this article focuses on techniques and results of corrective ankle arthrodesis for varus ankle OA with and without cavovarus foot and the possible concomitant procedures.

CAUSES AND BIOMECHANICS OF THE VARUS ANKLE AND HINDFOOT
Causes

Previous clinical and epidemiologic studies have identified that the most common cause for ankle OA is post-traumatic, with varus as the predominant malalignment.[2,8] The ankle joint is rarely affected by primary OA unlike the hip and knee joint. Saltzman and colleagues[8] evaluated 639 patients presenting with painful end-stage ankle OA; 70% of his cohort were classified as post-traumatic OA. Subgroup analysis of the post-traumatic ankle OA (445 patients) group showed rotational ankle fractures (164 patients) were the most common cause, followed by previous ligamental injuries (126 patients). In Valderrabano and coworkers' series of 390 consecutive patients (406 ankles) with painful end-stage ankle OA, 78% were classified as post-traumatic OA.[2] Subgroup analysis of the post-traumatic ankle OA (313 patients) group showed malleolar fractures (157 patients) as the most common cause, followed by ankle ligament lesions (60 patients), and tibial plafond fracture (58 patients). In a further series Valderrabano and coworkers[9] looked specifically at ligamentous post-traumatic ankle OA. Concomitant varus hindfoot deformity was found in 52% of the patients. Repetitive ankle sprains in sports (soccer, 33%) was the main cause of ligamentous post-traumatic ankle OA and 85% injured the lateral ankle ligaments.

The causes of the varus deformity can also be generally divided into bone deformities, chronic ligament insufficiency, muscle imbalance, or a combination of all. Neurologic diseases can play a major role in causing varus deformity. Initially, these pathologic conditions begin as correctable deformities, but, over time, they may become rigid, causing abnormal biomechanics of the foot and ankle and leading to secondary OA with fixed varus or cavovarus deformity. The possible causes of varus ankle OA are summarized in **Box 1**.

Biomechanics

Ankle varus and cavovarus deformities are caused by an abnormality in the hindfoot, midfoot, or forefoot. If the abnormality is in the hindfoot, as in patients with a chronic lateral ankle instability, the talus makes a pathologic internal rotation and anterior subluxation, and, over time, an asymmetric medial ankle OA. In such a situation, the hindfoot goes into varus and the forefoot goes into supination. With such an internally rotated foot deformity, the patient is not able to walk. Therefore, the forefoot tries to compensate this by making a metatarsus primus flexus by an overactivity of the peroneus longus muscle. In this way, while walking the patient has a hindfoot varus and a plantigrade forefoot. Over time, the posterior tibialis muscle overrides the peroneus brevis muscle and the whole system decompensates totally.

If the deformity is in the forefoot (eg, by an overpull of the peroneus longus muscle creating a plantarflexed first metatarsal), then the hindfoot is obliged to

Box 1
Causes of the varus ankle osteoarthritis
Post-Traumatic:
Varus malunion of tibial shaft fractures
Varus malunion of tibial plafond fractures
Varus malunion of talus and calcaneus fractures
Avascular necrosis of talus
Chronic lateral ankle ligament insufficiency
Post compartment syndrome
Congenital:
Residual clubfoot (talipes equinovarus)
Tarsal coalition
Excessive tibial external rotation
Neurologic:
Stroke
Central and peripheral nerve disorders
Hereditary motor sensory neuropathy/Charcot-Marie-Tooth disease
Polio
Cerebral palsy
Degenerative:
Rheumatoid osteoarthritis
Varus knee osteoarthritis
Charcot osteoarthropathy

go into inversion by the high midfoot arch (pes cavus). This leads to an inability of the foot to act as a shock absorber by limiting hindfoot eversion. Over time, the peroneus brevis muscle becomes weaker and the lateral ankle instability results in a varus ankle with secondary degeneration (degenerative pes cavovarus). Charcot-Marie-Tooth disease is a good example of this pathologic condition.

During the gait cycle for patients with a cavovarus deformity of the hindfoot, the subtalar joint is more vertical and the talar head tends to impinge on anterior process of the calcaneus, which results in less subtalar movement. Both subtalar and transverse tarsal joints are rigid, which diminishes the ability of the foot to work as a shock absorber during the early stage of the stance phase.[10,11] The center of pressure line of the foot is strongly lateralized.[11] In surface electromyographs analysis, an overfiring of the posterior tibialis muscle, peroneus longus muscle, and gastrocnemius medialis muscle are expected.

To achieve successful treatment of the varus ankle, recognition of the associated deformities is vital, that is, lateral chronic ankle instability, varus heel, hindfoot OA, overfiring of muscles (as posterior tibial muscle/peroneus longus), forefoot malalignment, lessor toes deformities, Achilles tendon tightness, knee deformities, and contralateral lower limb malalignment.

INDICATIONS FOR ANKLE ARTHRODESIS

In varus ankle OA, it is important to have a clear indication list for ankle arthrodesis to cleanly separate joint-preserving surgery and total ankle arthroplasty. The indications for an ankle arthrodesis in a varus ankle OA are:

- Physically heavily active manual laborer
- Severe varus deformity
- Severe ankle instability
- Previous ankle infection; however, no current signs for infection and/or osteomyelitis
- Insufficient bone stock/severe osteoporosis
- Advanced osteonecrosis of the talus
- Severe neuromuscular ankle/hindfoot deformities
- Charcot osteoarthropathy
- Inadequate soft tissue envelope

SURGICAL TECHNIQUES FOR ANKLE ARTHRODESIS AND NECESSARY SURGICAL PROCEDURES

The optimum alignment of arthrodesis is neutral flexion-extension, 0° to 5° of hindfoot valgus, 5° to 10° of external rotation, and 0 to 1 cm posterior displacement of the talus in relation to distal tibia to optimize the lever arm.[12–14] Following a well-positioned ankle arthrodesis, the energy expenditure required is 3% greater than for a normal counterpart, whereas the gait efficiency achieves 90% of normal at a similar pace of walking.[15] In severe varus ankle OA, it is important to correct the deformity perioperatively because varus malalignment is found to be a risk factor for nonunion after arthrodesis.[16] Varus malalignment locks the midfoot joints during normal heel rise and results in an inability to compensate through the midfoot, causing excess lateral forefoot weight bearing.[17]

Approaches for Ankle Arthrodesis

The possible approaches for ankle arthrodesis are the following: anterior ankle approach, lateral transfibular approach, combined lateral and medial mini-open arthrotomy approach, arthroscopic technique, or posterior approach. The most commonly used open approaches are the anterior and lateral transfibular approaches. The best approach should take into account the apex of the deformity and the integrity of the soft tissues and allow for an additional procedure if needed, either by extending the incision (extensile approach) or by placing a separate incision with a good skin bridge.

Anterior ankle approach

The anterior approach to the ankle is performed through the interval between tibialis anterior and extensor hallucis longus tendons. It is important to raise a thick skin flap to maintain vascularity and avoid injury to the neurovascular bundle, which runs between the extensor hallucis longus and the extensor digitorum longus. Before working on the joint surfaces, it is essential to rebalance the medial soft tissues: release of the deltoid ligament or even elongate the posterior tibial tendon. The joint arthrodesis surfaces are prepared either by flat cuts or subchondral cartilage removal. The flat cut technique consists of cutting the distal tibia and dome of the talus with the saw blade perpendicular to the axis of the tibia, which has a good bone exposure and healing; however, this surgical technique may result in substantial shortening of the extremity. Subchondral cartilage removal removes the cartilage by preserving the subchondral bone, thus maintaining the congruity of the ankle joint by keeping the height of the talus and preserving the length. This is followed by subchondral microfracturing with drills or guidewires. Cartilage removal techniques offer little opportunity for angular correction, whereas straight, flat cuts allow correction of significant deformity. In a varus ankle, the medial tibial plafond is usually eroded up to the sclerotic hard bare bone with incongruency. It is important to recognize and address this issue during joint preparation to prevent the arthrodesis going into a varus malunion or delayed union/ nonunion. A flat cut may help to avoid this issue. If a cartilage-removing technique was used, the medial defect should be grafted with autologous bone. In both subtechniques, it is important to remove the cartilage in the medial ankle gutter also, to get bone union at the medial ankle.

The prepared surfaces are brought together, with the talus shifted posteriorly and medially so that the anterior cut of the talus matches the anterior cut of the tibia. Joint position is secured with a compression clamp. Screw-K-wires are positioned with the help of fluoroscopy, and three cannulated compressing screws (7.0 CCS Compressing Screws, Medartis, Exton, PA) are inserted. The first screw trajectory runs from the posteromedial aspect of the tibia toward the neck of talus, whereas the K-wire here is placed by a percutaneous incision at the posteromedial supramalleolar aspect of the tibia. The second screw is placed percutaneously from the posterolateral aspect of the tibia to the anterior talar neck, and the third screw increases the rigidity from the anterior tibia to the posterior talar body. All three screws should never cross altogether at the arthrodesis joint line. Biomechanical studies have shown that a three-screws fixation technique was significantly better than two-screws in a crossed configuration and the recommended fixation is one screw medially, one laterally, and one anterior from the tibia to the talus.[18] However, excellent clinical results for the anterior approach have been reported with a two-screw technique placed from the medial tibia into the posteromedial and anterolateral talar head and also a four-screw technique (two screws parallel from the anterior aspect of the distal tibia into the body of the talus, one posteromedial into the anterolateral portion of the talar head, and the fourth screw percutaneously from the posterolateral aspect of the distal fibula approximately 1.5 cm proximal to the tip of the lateral malleolus into the dorsal portion of the talar body).[19,20]

An alternative fixation method of the anterior ankle arthrodesis could also use an anterior, anatomically preshaped tibial plate.[21]

Lateral transfibular approach

In the lateral transfibular approach, the skin incision starts 10 cm proximal to the tip of fibula curving toward the base of the fourth metatarsal bone.[22,23] A full-thickness flap is developed along the wound incision. Using an oscillating saw, the fibula is transected obliquely 2 cm above the joint line and posteriorly rotated. The medial third of the fibula is removed, exposing the cancellous bone to be used at the end as a lateral onlay buttress graft to the ankle arthrodesis. The excised medial third fragment is kept and used as autologous bone graft.

If the varus deformity is not correctable, a medial incision is made 4 cm over the anteromedial aspect of medial malleolus. The soft tissue is dissected anteriorly and posterior-medially with protection of deltoid ligament. The medial malleolus can be shortened to facilitate the realignment.

The fixation method can also be performed with three compression screws or with an anterior plate. The distal fibula is then added as a natural lateral bony "plate" fixed by two cortical screws.

Combined lateral and medial mini-open arthrotomy approach

The minimally invasive or mini-open arthrotomy approach popularized by Myerson tries to combine the advantages of the open and arthroscopic ankle arthrodesis methods while limiting their respective disadvantages.[24,25] Two 2- to 3-cm vertical incisions are centered over the standard portal sites for ankle arthroscopy. The anteromedial incision is made immediately medial to the tibialis anterior tendon, between the tendon and the notch of the medial malleolus, whereas the anterolateral incision is made in the space between the lateral border of the peroneus tertius tendon and the anterior border of the fibula. The joint surfaces are prepared through these incisions with curettes and chisels with the aid of laminar spreaders or K-wire-distractors. No motorized burrs are used to limit potential thermal necrosis of the bone that may lead to delayed union or nonunion of the arthrodesis. The fixation method is similar to the anterior ankle approach with percutaneous compressing screws. The combined lateral and medial mini-open arthrotomy approach is best used in cases without significant deformity or bone loss.

Arthroscopic Technique

Arthroscopic ankle arthrodesis is gaining in popularity because of its perceived benefits, such as decreased incision size to minimize morbidity, shorter hospital stay, shorter time to union with similar, or better union rates.[26] Standard anteromedial and anterolateral arthroscopic portals are used. The joint surfaces are prepared with motorized burr, abraider, and curettes. Rigid fixation is achieved with percutaneous cannulated compressing screws. This technique is good for cases with minimal or no deformity or bone loss. However, the authors do not recommend it in moderate to severe varus deformity, although some would argue otherwise. The results of this are further discussed later.

Posterior Approach

The posterior approach is used as salvage procedure, especially for revision cases. In such cases, it is often performed as a tibio-talar-calcaneal (TTC) arthrodesis.[27]

Concomitant Procedures Apart from Ankle Arthrodesis

In subtalar varus deformity without subtalar OA, a lateral displacement calcaneal osteotomy is added to correct the pulling vector of the Achilles tendon, which becomes more medialized with varus hindfoot deformity. A 4-cm oblique incision is made laterally over the calcaneus, anterior to the Achilles tendon insertion, from the posterior superior tuberosity to the anteroinferior tuberosity. A subperiosteal dissection is made in line with the incision, and a transverse osteotomy is performed from lateral to medial across both cortices, perpendicular to the long axis of the calcaneus, with a large oscillating saw. The posterior fragment is then translated laterally 5 to 10 mm until the heel is in physiologic valgus and fixed with two cannulated compressing screws (CCS Screws, Medartis; **Fig. 1**).

In subtalar varus deformity with OA, a TTC arthrodesis is indicated. TTC arthrodesis is performed with a medial incision for soft tissue release of the tight medial structures and a lateral transfibular incision as described previously but extended distally to gain access to the subtalar joint. The joint surfaces are prepared with an oscillating saw to make two parallel cuts at the ankle joint. Following removal of residual articular cartilage in the subtalar joint, several fixation techniques are used. Options include a pure multiple cannulated screws construct, a plantar retrograde hindfoot nail with or without fibular onlay graft, or a TTC plate fixation[28] This surgery can also be performed

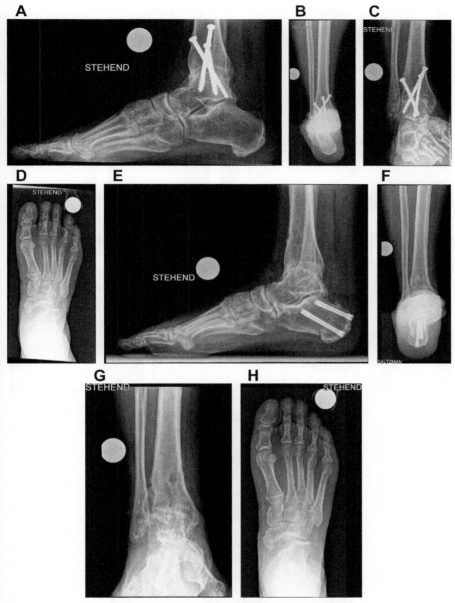

Fig. 1. Lateral sliding calcaneal osteotomy after ankle arthrodesis. (*A–D*) Preoperative radiographs. (*E–H*) Postoperative radiographs. Besides the hardware removal of the ankle arthrodesis, a lateral sliding calcaneal osteotomy has been performed to realign the hindfoot.

by an anterior approach to prepare the ankle joint in combination with a limited sinus tarsi incision to prepare the subtalar joint or through a posterior approach.

In talonavicular joint OA and deformity with ankle and subtalar disease, a pantalar arthrodesis is indicated (**Fig. 2**). It is described as a fusion of the three joints around

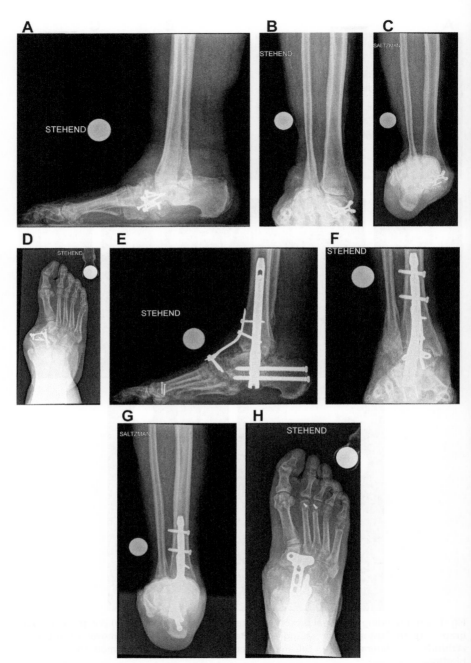

Fig. 2. Pantalar arthrodesis. This case is a valgus and not a varus ankle case, but properly depicts the pantalar arthrodesis technique. (*A–D*) Preoperative radiographs. (*E–H*) Postoperative radiographs.

the talus: the tibiotalar, subtalar, and Chopart joint. This procedure starts with a patient placed on the supine position with a bump supporting the ipsilateral buttock and maintaining the internal rotation of the foot. An extended lateral position is used over the lateral malleolus, and the fibula is osteotomized 2 cm proximal to joint line after stripping off the soft tissue, which is later used as an onlay graft to supplement the fusion (see transfibular approach). The ankle joint is debrided and reduced in neutral dorsiflexion and a five-degree external rotation; a hindfoot retrograde nail (HAN Nail, Depuy-Synthes, West Chester, PA) is then integrated. An anterior plate is then placed across the tibia and talus to the navicular bone after preparing the Chopart joint. Gastrocnemius recession (Strayer) is done if the Achilles tendon is tight. Finally, if needed, the calcaneocuboid joint is stabilized with a 5.0-mm cannulated CCS screw (CCS screw, Medartis).

In forefoot driven hindfoot varus (pes cavovarus) with varus ankle OA, beside the ankle arthrodesis, a dorsal closing wedge metatarsal osteotomy or reversed Cotton osteotomy at the medial cuneiform with planter fascia release are added to correct the whole deformity. Sometimes a lateral sliding calcaneal osteotomy might be needed to delay the onset of subtalar OA. Furthermore, a peroneus longus to brevis tendon transfer might be needed to reduce the plantarflexion force of the first ray. On the medial side, the contracted posterior tibialis tendon and the deltoid/spring ligament might need to be addressed: the posterior tibialis tendon elongated by z-shaped lengthening and the release of deltoid/spring ligament.

An overview of the additional possible surgeries by/after ankle arthrodesis are depicted in **Table 1**.

AFTER-TREATMENT

Postoperatively, the leg is kept in a splint and the patient is bedbound. The patient remains 15 kg partial weight bearing for 8 weeks in a walker (Aircast Walker Elite, DJO Global, Dallas, TX). Stitches are removed 2 weeks postoperative. If radiographs at 8 weeks show good evidence of healing, the patient is allowed to start full weight bearing according to their pain with shoes with a rocker-bottom-sole.

RESULTS

The outcome following varus ankle OA arthrodesis in the literature is sparse. We have summarized the results in **Table 2**. In most of the papers, we were not able to solely

Table 1
Summary of associated deformities and further procedure required in addition to ankle arthrodesis

Associated Deformities	Further Procedure Required in Addition to Ankle Arthrodesis
Varus hindfoot with no subtalar OA	Lateral sliding calcaneal OT/Dwyer calcaneal OT
Varus hindfoot with subtalar OA	Valgusating subtalar arthrodesis after ankle AD or primary tibio-talo-calcaneal AD
Pantalar OA	Pantalar AD
Tight gastroc-soleus complex	Strayer or proximal gastrocnemius recession
High arch (cavus)	Reversed Cotton ± plantar fascia release
Plantar flexed first metatarsal	Dorsal closing wedge first metatarsal osteotomy
Plantar flexed first metatarsal with overdrive of peroneal longus tendon	Dorsal closing wedge first metatarsal osteotomy and peroneal longus to brevis tendon transfer

Abbreviations: AD, arthrodesis; OT, osteotomy.

Table 2
Literature review of studies with open arthrodesis cases and long follow-up

Author	Duration	Number of Cases	Follow-up	Technique	Fixation Method	Outcome	Fusion Time	Fusion Rate	Non union	Delayed Union	Infection	Permanent Implant	Arthritis of Other Joints
Ferkel and Hewitt,[39] 2005	July 1989–December 2002	35 patients	72 mo	Arthroscopic arthrodesis	2 or 3 screws	By Morgan system 29 (83%) good to excellent, 5 (14%) fair result, 1 (3%) poor result	11.8 wk	97%	1 (2.8%)	3 (8.5%)	0 (0%)	11 (31.4%)	0%
Smith and Wood,[29] 2007	October 2001–June 2004	25 ankles in 23 patients	22 mo	Open arthrodesis (anterior approach)	2 parallel screws	Mean AOFAS function score before operation was 25.5 (11–39), improving to 43.7 (31–58) at follow-up	11.4 wk	97%	1 (4%)	0%	0%	0%	0%
Schmid et al,[35] 2017	2005–2012	35 patients	48 mo	Open arthrodesis transfibular approach and additional anteromedial incision/direct anterior approach	2 or 3 partially threaded 6.5-mm cannulated screws	Ankle Osteoarthritis Scale mean, 33.9; 95% CI, 17.8–49.9 Ankle Arthritis Scale mean, 27.2; 95% CI, 19.7–35.2	N/A	97%	1 (3%)	0%	0%	5 (14%)	0%

Study	Period	Patients	Follow-up	Technique	Fixation	AOFAS						
Al-Ashhab,[40] 2017	December 2010–December 2014	20 patents tibial pilon fractures	34 mo	Open arthrodesis direct transfibular approach	Retrograde calcaneal nail	AOFAS ankle score mean, 85.4 (range, 80–86) at final follow-up	16 wk	100%	0%	0%	0%	0%	0%
Nielsen et al,[41] 2008	1994–2005	48 patients	12 mo	Ankle arthrodesis performed with open surgery technique through direct transfibular approach	2 percutaneous screws (usually the diameter of 7.5 mm)	N/A	12 wk	84%	8 (16%) 0%	8 (16%)	4 (8%)	8 (16%)	0%

Abbreviations: AOFAS, American Orthopedic Foot and Ankle function score; CI, confidence interval; N/A, not applicable.
The studies showed good fusion rates and satisfactory outcomes on different scoring system with acceptable complication rate.

isolate the series into varus OA arthrodesis. Many papers consider coronal deformity of varus and valgus as the same entity even though they are of a different biomechanical pathologic process.

Open Arthrodesis Related to Varus Osteoarthritis

Smith and Wood[29] reported a consecutive series of 23 patients (25 ankles) who had OA of the ankle with severe varus or valgus deformity (defined as more than 20°) and were treated by open arthrodesis through an anterior approach using two parallel medial compression screw configurations primarily. In this series, 20 ankles had severe varus deformity of an average of 28° (range, 20–45). Of these 20 varus ankles, 13 required a resection osteotomy of the lateral malleolus to allow correction of the deformity and union of the fibular osteotomy occurred in all instances. In two cases where the skin was adherent to the malleolus, the osteotomy had to be achieved through a separate lateral incision. Four patients had a fixed plantar flexion deformity of the first ray and a proximal dorsiflexion osteotomy of the first metatarsal was then carried out. The mean American Orthopedic Foot and Ankle function score before operation was 25.5 (11–39), improving to 43.7 (31–58) at follow-up. There was one nonunion (varus of 20°, bilateral sequential fusion) in this series and this was successfully revised with bone grafting. All the cases corrected to within 5° of neutral. Fortin and coworkers[30] reported six patients (eight cavovarus feet) who had end-stage varus OA (Takakura stage 3) who underwent arthrodesis, of which three feet required a dorsiflexion osteotomy of the first metatarsal. All had an improvement in functional scores. The hindfoot alignment improved in all but one patient, who had slight residual varus. Saltzman's center reviewed all their uncomplicated primary open ankle fusions conducted at their institution over an 11-year period (215 open ankle fusion, 209 patients) to identify factors influencing operative outcomes.[31] These cases were treated by a variety of approaches and arthrodesis techniques. Their overall union rate was 91%. They found that nonunion was three times more likely to occur after a previous subtalar fusion, and two times more likely to occur in patients with preoperative varus ankle alignment.

Arthroscopic Ankle Arthrodesis Related to Varus Osteoarthritis

There are several papers looking at the effects of preoperative deformity on arthroscopic ankle arthrodesis. Winson and colleagues[32] reported a consecutive series of 116 patients (118 ankles) who had an arthroscopic ankle arthrodesis with a coronal-plane deformity ranging from 22 valgus to 28 varus, but most (94 cases) were within 10° varus/valgus. The mean time to union was 12 weeks (6–20), whereas nonunion occurred in nine cases (7.6%). Four cases required intraoperative calcaneal osteotomy to realign the hindfoot. In their series Gougoulias and coworkers[33] subdivided his cohort into two groups; minor coronal-plane deformity with a varus or valgus deformity of less than 15° (48 patients, 5.6° ± 2.9°) and a major deformity with a varus or valgus deformity of more than 15° (30 patients, 24.7° ± 7.5°). In the group with a major deformity, a further debridement of the tibial surface was performed to correct the deformity. Four patients in the major deformity group required concomitant subtalar arthrodesis. Their overall fusion rate is 97%. There was no significant difference between both groups in terms of nonunion rates (one in each group), time to union (13.1 vs 11.6 weeks), clinical outcomes, and complications. In both groups, good postoperative frontal alignment correction was achieved (0.7° valgus vs 0.4° valgus). Dannawi and colleagues[34] reviewed their cohort of 55 patients who had arthroscopic ankle arthrodesis and divided them into two groups like Gougoulias and coworkers: minor coronal-plane deformity (n = 31) and major deformity (n = 24). The overall fusion rate was 91%. There was no difference in the union rates and Mazur ankle grading system between both groups but the group with a coronal deformity of equal to or more than 15° had a significantly longer mean time of union (12.7 weeks vs 8.8 weeks). Both authors concluded that arthroscopic ankle arthrodesis is appropriate and advocate its use in patients who have ankle OA with a marked deformity.

The Canadian Orthopedic Foot and Ankle Society study group looked at the effect of preoperative deformity on arthroscopic and open ankle fusion.[35] Preoperative deformity was the same regarding sagittal alignment and overall coronal alignment, but the arthroscopic group had less tibial deformity (tibial plafond angle range 0–19° vs 0–43°). In terms of clinical outcome, they found that preoperative deformity in the coronal or the sagittal plane did not affect the Ankle Osteoarthritis Scale and the Ankle Arthritis Score at final follow-up. The radiologic outcome at 12 months after surgery was identical in both groups, with proper alignment in the coronal plane (medial tibiotalar angle 89.3° vs 88.3°) and sagittal plane alignment regarding lateral talar station (1.3 mm vs 2.3 mm) and lateral tibiotalar angle (111.2° vs 110.4°). They concluded that arthroscopic and open ankle fusion yielded equivalent results for patient-reported outcome measures and radiographic alignment in patients with coronal and sagittal joint deformity.

After the surgical intervention, patients usually have normal gait pattern and decrease the use of walking stick. Few patients improve their ability to ascend and descend the stairs. However, detailed gait analysis reveals decreased walking speed secondary to a shortened stride length; this might be caused by the loss of 60% to 70% from the sagittal plane motion; this loss of motion is frequently compensated by an increase in transverse tarsal and midfoot motion. Fortunately, the gait is improved with shoe modification by adding a rocker bottom sole or shock-absorbing solid ankle cushion heel, and, even without modified shoes, gait remains efficient.

In a 22-year longitudinal study on ankle arthrodesis, the results showed an increased incidence of ipsilateral foot (but not knee) arthritis in patients who previously underwent successful ankle arthrodesis, which consequently limited the patient's function.[36] For this reason, the treating surgeon must adapt to address more complex types of ankle arthritis effectively by performing a TTC, pantalar, or TC fusion rather than a strict ankle joint fusion.

DISCUSSION

Ankle arthrodesis is the most common surgical treatment of end-stage varus ankle OA if nonoperative management has failed. Nevertheless, there are various other surgical options for treating ankle OA, which include joint-preserving surgery and total ankle arthroplasty.[37] Patient factors, severity of the deformity, and extent of the OA influence the decision-making process.

In the early stages of varus ankle OA with reasonably well-preserved cartilage, the optimal choice of treatment is to shift intra-articular load and stresses from medially to laterally by an osteotomy.[3] Careful evaluation of the underlying deformity as being supramalleolar, subtalar, or a combination allows the surgeon to reduce the risk of the osteotomy failing. Additionally, this procedure might be delayed or obviated by the need for ankle arthrodesis or arthroplasty.

Advances in total ankle arthroplasty designs have challenged the perception that ankle arthrodesis is the treatment of choice for ankle OA.[38] The preservation of ankle range of motion, gait improvement, and stress reduction on the subtalar and Chopart joints in total ankle arthroplasty are perceived advantages over ankle arthrodesis. The ideal indication for ankle arthroplasty is older age (>50 year old), low activity level, little or no associated deformity, and accepted ankle range of motion. Patients with degenerative or previous fusions of the adjacent joints or bilateral ankle OA are also considered good candidates for ankle arthroplasty. Soft tissue and bone stock are also critical in influencing the choice of surgical decision.

If a young patient presents with severe ankle deformity, traumatic bone loss, osteoporosis, obesity, stiff joint, or a history of previous infections, the treatment of choice is ankle arthrodesis. Absolute contraindications for ankle arthroplasty are Charcot arthropathy and vascular or neurologic insufficiency, and patients with these conditions are good candidates for ankle arthrodesis. In most postoperative ankle arthrodesis, the surgical outcomes are good to excellent if ideal indications are present and the surgery is performed with rigid fixation and addresses associated deformities.

Careful clinical evaluation and detailed radiographic studies are essential to select optimal surgical options and to achieve excellent surgical outcome. Understanding the underlying causes of varus ankle OA and progression of the deformity is crucial to choosing the best surgical option and achieving a satisfactory result. Ankle arthrodesis is a technically demanding surgical procedure that is frequently associated with complications, such as nonunion. Thus, patients should be screened for modifiable risk factors of arthrodesis nonunion.

SUMMARY

Varus ankle OA has multiple underlying causes that can contribute to this complex pathologic entity. Recognition of associated deformities is vital. Although corrective ankle arthrodesis is the gold standard treatment of end-stage ankle OA with varus deformity, this procedure presents a significant surgical challenge and is only indicated if nonoperative treatment failed to relieve the pain and stiffness.

Different surgical approaches are used and the best one should be one that allows for additional procedures to be performed safely if needed. The surgeon's experience and careful preoperatively assessment of the associated deformities present should guide choosing the right approach. In severe varus cases, bony procedures might need to be combined with soft tissue realignment procedure to restore a more normal mechanical axis.

The main complication of ankle arthrodesis is nonunion. However, modifying risk factors, careful preoperative planning, and meticulous operative technique all contribute to a successful outcome.

ACKNOWLEDGMENTS

As only 2 maximal authors could be listed for this article, we would like to thank the following colleagues for their contribution: Saud Alshalawi, Kar Hao Teoh, Alexej Barg, Yousef Alrashidi, Ahmed Galhoum, Martin Wiewiorski, Mario Herrera.

REFERENCES

1. Ahn T-K, Yi Y, Cho J-H, et al. A cohort study of patients undergoing distal tibial osteotomy without fibular osteotomy for medial ankle arthritis with mortise widening. J Bone Joint Surg Am 2015;97(5):381–8.
2. Valderrabano V, Horisberger M, Russell I, et al. Etiology of ankle osteoarthritis. Clin Orthop Relat Res 2009;467(7):1800–6.
3. Stufkens SA, van Bergen CJ, Blankevoort L, et al. The role of the fibula in varus and valgus deformity of the tibia: a biomechanical study. J Bone Joint Surg Br 2011;93(9):1232–9.

4. Horn DM, Fragomen AT, Rozbruch SR. Supramalleolar osteotomy using circular external fixation with six-axis deformity correction of the distal tibia. Foot Ankle Int 2011;32(10):986–93.
5. Takakura Y, Tanaka Y, Kumai T, et al. Low tibial osteotomy for osteoarthritis of the ankle. Results of a new operation in 18 patients. J Bone Joint Surg Br 1995;77(1):50–4.
6. Kim J-B, Yi Y, Kim J-Y, et al. Weight-bearing computed tomography findings in varus ankle osteoarthritis: abnormal internal rotation of the talus in the axial plane. Skeletal Radiol 2017;46(8):1071–80.
7. Abidi NA, Gruen GS, Conti SF. Ankle arthrodesis: indications and techniques. J Am Acad Orthop Surg 2000;8(3):200–9.
8. Saltzman CL, Salamon ML, Blanchard GM, et al. Epidemiology of ankle arthritis: report of a consecutive series of 639 patients from a tertiary orthopaedic center. Iowa Orthop J 2005;25:44–6.
9. Valderrabano V, Hintermann B, Horisberger M, et al. Ligamentous posttraumatic ankle osteoarthritis. Am J Sports Med 2006;34(4):612–20.
10. Apostle KL, Sangeorzan BJ. Anatomy of the varus foot and ankle. Foot Ankle Clin 2012;17(1):1–11.
11. Chilvers M, Manoli A 2nd. The subtle cavus foot and association with ankle instability and lateral foot overload. Foot Ankle Clin 2008;13(2):315–24, vii.
12. Buck P, Morrey BF, Chao EY. The optimum position of arthrodesis of the ankle. A gait study of the knee and ankle. J Bone Joint Surg Am 1987;69(7):1052–62.
13. Hefti FL, Baumann JU, Morscher EW. Ankle joint fusion: determination of optimal position by gait analysis. Arch Orthop Trauma Surg 1980;96(3):187–95.
14. Thomas RH, Daniels TR. Ankle arthritis. J Bone Joint Surg Am 2003;85-A(5):923–36.
15. Waters RL, Barnes G, Husserl T, et al. Comparable energy expenditure after arthrodesis of the hip and ankle. J Bone Joint Surg Am 1988;70(7):1032–7.
16. Scranton PEJ, Fu FH, Brown TD. Ankle arthrodesis: a comparative clinical and biomechanical evaluation. Clin Orthop Relat Res 1980;151:234–43.
17. Muir DC, Amendola A, Saltzman CL. Long-term outcome of ankle arthrodesis. Foot Ankle Clin N Am 2002;7:703–8.
18. Ogilvie-Harris DJ, Fitsialos D, Hedman TP. Arthrodesis of the ankle. A comparison of two versus three screw fixation in a crossed configuration. Clin Orthop Relat Res 1994;(304):195–9.
19. Zwipp H, Rammelt S, Endres T, et al. High union rates and function scores at midterm followup with ankle arthrodesis using a four screw technique. Clin Orthop Relat Res 2010;468(4):958–68.
20. Gordon D, Zicker R, Cullen N, et al. Open ankle arthrodeses via an anterior approach. Foot Ankle Int 2013;34(3):386–91.
21. Wiewiorski M, Barg A, Schlemmer T, et al. Ankle joint fusion with an anatomically preshaped anterior locking plate. J Foot Ankle Surg 2016;55(2):414–7.
22. ADAMS JC. Arthrodesis of the ankle joint; experiences with the transfibular approach. J Bone Joint Surg Br 1948;30B(3):506–11.
23. Mann RA, Van Manen JW, Wapner K, et al. Ankle fusion. Clin Orthop Relat Res 1991;268:49–55.
24. Paremain GD, Miller SD, Myerson MS. Ankle arthrodesis: results after the miniarthrotomy technique. Foot Ankle Int 1996;17(5):247–52.
25. Miller SD, Paremain GP, Myerson MS. The miniarthrotomy technique of ankle arthrodesis: a cadaver study of operative vascular compromise and early clinical results. Orthopedics 1996;19(5):425–30.

26. Elmlund AO, Winson IG. Arthroscopic ankle arthrodesis. Foot Ankle Clin 2015; 20(1):71–80.

27. Pellegrini MJ, Schiff AP, Adams SBJ, et al. Outcomes of tibiotalocalcaneal arthrodesis through a posterior Achilles tendon-splitting approach. Foot Ankle Int 2016;37(3):312–9.

28. Shah KS, Younger AS. Primary tibiotalocalcaneal arthrodesis. Foot Ankle Clin 2011;16(1):115–36.

29. Smith R, Wood PL. Arthrodesis of the ankle in the presence of a large deformity in the coronal plane. J Bone Joint Surg Br 2007;89-B(5):615–9.

30. Fortin PT, Guettler J, Manoli A 2nd. Idiopathic cavovarus and lateral ankle instability: recognition and treatment implications relating to ankle arthritis. Foot Ankle Int 2002;23(11):1031–7.

31. Chalayon O, Wang B, Blankenhorn B, et al. Factors affecting the outcomes of uncomplicated primary open ankle arthrodesis. Foot Ankle Int 2015;36(10):1170–9.

32. Winson IG, Robinson DE, Allen PE. Arthroscopic ankle arthrodesis. J Bone Joint Surg Br 2005;87(3):343–7.

33. Gougoulias NE, Agathangelidis FG, Parsons SW. Arthroscopic ankle arthrodesis. Foot Ankle Int 2007;28(6):695–706.

34. Dannawi Z, Nawabi DH, Patel A, et al. Arthroscopic ankle arthrodesis: are results reproducible irrespective of pre-operative deformity? Foot Ankle Surg 2011;17(4): 294–9.

35. Schmid T, Krause F, Penner MJ, et al. Effect of preoperative deformity on arthroscopic and open ankle fusion outcomes. Foot Ankle Int 2017;38(12):1301–10.

36. Coester LM, Saltzman CL, Leupold J, et al. Long-term results following ankle arthrodesis for post-traumatic arthritis. J Bone Joint Surg Am 2001;83-A(2): 219–28.

37. Easley ME. Surgical treatment of the arthritic varus ankle. Foot Ankle Clin 2012; 17(4):665–86.

38. Morash J, Walton DM, Glazebrook M. Ankle arthrodesis versus total ankle arthroplasty. Foot Ankle Clin 2017;22(2):251–66.

39. Ferkel RD, Hewitt M. Long-term results of arthroscopic ankle arthrodesis. Foot Ankle Int 2005;26(4):275–80.

40. Al-Ashhab ME. Primary ankle arthrodesis for severely comminuted tibial pilon fractures. Orthopedics 2017;40(2):e378–81.

41. Nielsen KK, Linde F, Jensen NC. The outcome of arthroscopic and open surgery ankle arthrodesis: a comparative retrospective study on 107 patients. Foot Ankle Surg 2008;14(3):153–7.

Two-Stage Varus Correction

Brian Steginsky, DO[a], Steven L. Haddad, MD[b],*

KEYWORDS

- Cavovarus • Varus deformity • Tibiotalar deformity • Total ankle arthroplasty
- Revision total ankle arthroplasty

KEY POINTS

- Coronal plane deformity following total ankle arthroplasty has been associated with poor clinical outcomes and early prosthesis failure.
- Neutral mechanical alignment and prosthetic joint stability must be achieved through meticulous surgical planning and precise technical execution.
- Cavovarus foot deformity and varus malalignment of the lower extremity is reviewed, with particular emphasis as it relates to total ankle arthroplasty.
- Correction of varus malalignment may be performed at the time of total ankle arthroplasty or as a 2-stage procedure.
- Surgeon experience, revision total ankle arthroplasty, and subtalar arthrodesis should be considerations when contemplating 2-stage varus correction.

Total ankle arthroplasty (TAA) has gained popularity as an alternative treatment to ankle arthrodesis for end-stage ankle arthritis. Advancing technology and improved prosthetic designs have led to better clinical outcomes, resulting in a renewed interest in TAA among orthopedic foot and ankle surgeons. However, the procedure remains relatively new compared with hip and knee arthroplasty, which has demonstrated superior longevity spanning several more decades.[1–4] Most of our understanding of TAA has been extrapolated from principles first established in hip and knee arthroplasty.

The basic principles of total joint arthroplasty, regardless of type, are to achieve neutral mechanical alignment and prosthetic joint stability.[5,6] Malalignment and prosthetic joint instability result in edge wear, accelerated polyethylene wear, and early component failure.[5–9] Coronal plane deformity following TAA has been associated with poor clinical outcomes and early prosthesis failure.[10,11] Historically, preoperative coronal plane deformity greater than 15° was considered a contraindication to TAA.[10,11] However, more recent literature has demonstrated that clinical outcomes

Disclosure Statement: Dr B. Steginsky: Nothing to disclose. S.L. Haddad: Royalty Bearing Surgeon, Wright Medical Technology, Inc.; Consultant, Wright Medical Technology, Inc.
[a] OhioHealth Orthopedic Surgeons, 303 East Town Street, Columbus, OH 43215, USA; [b] Illinois Bone and Joint Institute, LLC, 2401 Ravine Way, Glenview, IL 60025, USA
* Corresponding author.
E-mail address: slhaddadmd@gmail.com

are independent of preoperative tibiotalar alignment when mechanical alignment is restored to neutral.[12] We do not believe that there is a contraindication to TAA in the presence of large preoperative coronal plane deformity if neutral mechanical alignment can be achieved during surgery.

Cavovarus foot deformity and varus malalignment of the lower extremity is reviewed, with particular attention as it relates to TAA. Indications and surgical technique for the correction of 2-stage varus deformities is also discussed.

CLINICAL EVALUATION

It is critical that the surgeon performs a through clinical evaluation and workup. Preoperative assessment must include identification and management of all modifiable risk factors. We perform serum nicotine testing 1 month before surgery, and repeat the test 1 week before surgery to confirm complete nicotine abstinence. Preoperative consultation with a vascular surgeon is indicated for any patient with a history or presentation of vascular insufficiency. If the patient had previous foot and ankle surgery, the operative reports should be obtained and reviewed. An attempt should be made to use any previous surgical scars and maintain adequate skin bridges to minimize the risk of wound necrosis. Consultation with a plastic surgeon may be appropriate if there is an anticipated risk of postoperative wound complications. We have implemented a postsurgical compression wrap protocol to lower incision complications by decreasing the tension of edema on these sites.[13,14] Recently, we have expanded our indications to include preoperative compression wrapping for patients with venous stasis and chronic lower extremity edema, especially those undergoing staged reconstructive TAA.

The surgeon must perform a through history to identify any contraindications to TAA. All general contraindications to total joint arthroplasty are applicable (ie, history of deep infection), but particular attention must be given to potential neuromuscular diseases that may preclude TAA. Neuromuscular diseases might manifest as foot and ankle disorders through neuromuscular imbalance and eventual rigid foot malalignment. Spinal cord and peripheral nerve injuries, Charcot-Marie Tooth disease, and cerebral palsy may be excluded for TAA, but not always. Careful neurologic assessment must be performed to identify any motor or sensory deficits. Referral to neurology or genetic counseling should be considered if any concerns arise. Peripheral nerve injuries may undergo tendon transfer procedures to eliminate foot drop and other confounding factors that would otherwise preclude TAA. Charcot-Marie-Tooth may require similar tendon transfers, or various foot arthrodeses to provide a more permanent stable construct as a base for the TAA. As such, neuromuscular conditions should be evaluated on a case-by-case basis, using sound clinical judgment to predict the potential for TAA to relieve disabling ankle arthritis.

The mechanical alignment of the entire lower extremity must be evaluated. Deformity in the tibia leads to increased shear stress through the tibiotalar joint, which becomes increasingly more pronounced as the deformity occurs at more distal levels in both the coronal and sagittal planes.[15] We obtain full-length weight-bearing bilateral lower extremity radiographs to screen for deformity. Deformity is often multiplanar, and weight-bearing computed tomography (CT) scan may be helpful for preoperative planning.

The lateral ankle ligament complex and peroneal tendons should be carefully examined, as lateral ankle pathology is frequently implicated in cavovarus deformities. MRI is useful for evaluation; however, it is associated with a high rate of false positive results for peroneal tendon tears and only provides a static assessment of the lateral ankle soft tissue restraints.[16] In our practice, we preferentially use ultrasound, as it provides both static and dynamic assessment of the soft tissues. We believe dynamic assessment is useful to determine the degree of ligamentous attenuation and both the need for and magnitude of lateral ligament reconstruction.

Gait assessment is equally critical to fully appreciate any underlying muscular imbalance. Observation should be performed with the patient preferably in shorts (or, if that is not possible, with pant-legs rolled up past the knees) to allow for full limb assessment. Severe genu varum is often associated with varus thrust with gait as the posterolateral structures of the knee are often attenuated. Such eccentric loading about the ankle can result in increased stress to the medial compartment of the ankle joint, and potential medial component subsidence or late medial malleolar fracture if not addressed.

The foot and ankle should be examined with the patient standing, making it easier to identify any functional lateral ankle instability (**Fig. 1**A, B). We use a goniometer to measure the degree of hindfoot varus. The rigidity of the deformity should be evaluated by attempting to correct the hindfoot to neutral. If the hindfoot is rigid, then at the very least a realignment calcaneal osteotomy is appropriate. Radiographs must be reviewed carefully in rigid varus deformity, for often the calcaneus is shifted medially on the talus, creating further varus loading. Under these circumstances, subtalar arthrodesis requires not only a closing-wedge component, but lateral shift to redistribute the axis of weight-bearing to neutral.

Comprehensive weight-bearing radiographic series includes 5 views of the ankle (anteroposterior [AP], mortise, lateral, flexion, and extension), 2 views of the foot, and an axial heel alignment view.[17] Weight-bearing CT is useful to supplement plain radiographs.

The primary objective is to establish a plantigrade weight-bearing surface with complete correction (removal) of any varus deformity (whether in the tibia, ankle, or foot) in preparation for a second-stage TAA.

Genu Varum

Proximal malalignment should be corrected before performing a TAA. Deformity that occurs at the level of the proximal tibia (ie, genu varum) and is greater than 10° should be corrected with a total knee arthroplasty or high tibial osteotomy. We recommend waiting at least 4 months to allow postsurgical edema to resolve and to encourage full rehabilitation before undergoing a subsequent surgery. Furthermore, in complex staged deformity correction, we often restrict weight bearing for 6 weeks following TAA to minimize shearing forces through the tibiotalar joint and promote bony ingrowth of the metal prosthesis in potentially compromised bone. As such, our postoperative weight-bearing protocol after TAA interferes with the immediate weight-bearing goals following total knee arthroplasty.

Supramalleolar Tibia Varus

Tibial osteotomy should be considered when deformity is present in the midshaft of the tibia or supramalleolar region. The tibial osteotomy should be performed at the center of rotation of angulation to obviate the need for translational correction that may alter the axial loading on the ankle prosthesis. The surgical approach and hardware placement is particularly important when the correction is performed at the level of the distal tibia. It is important to plan both stages before performing the osteotomy to ensure that there are no unforeseen issues related to hardware placement during the second-stage TAA.

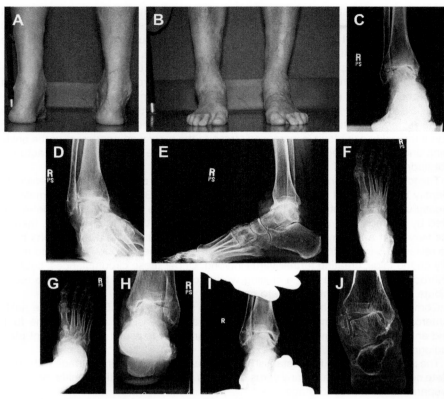

Fig. 1. Clinical photographs of a 65-year-old man who presented to the office with a severe varus deformity of the right ankle (*A*, *B*). Preoperative weight-bearing ankle radiographs demonstrate a severe incongruent varus tibiotalar deformity of 29° (*C–E*). Severe lateral ligament attenuation and subsequent varus talar tilt is noted. The longstanding tibiotalar incongruence resulted in erosion of the medial tibial plafond, medial gutter impingement (with deltoid ligament contracture), and osteophyte formation in the lateral joint space. AP and oblique weight-bearing foot radiographs demonstrate rotational deformity of the foot (*F, G*). Axial heel alignment radiograph demonstrates the varus position of the calcaneal tuberosity (*H*). We obtain reverse stress radiographs in the office to determine the reducibility of the deformity. In this particular case, the tibiotalar deformity is rigid as demonstrated with reverse stress radiographs (*I*). Coronal weight-bearing CT scan demonstrates a large osteophyte in the lateral joint space that will impede reduction of the talus, unless an aggressive lateral gutter and joint space debridement is performed at the time of surgery. The medial facet of the talus is impinging on the medial malleolus, resulting in osteophyte formation and deltoid ligament contracture (*J*).

Congruent Varus Tibiotalar Deformity

Congruent varus ankle deformity can often be corrected at the time of TAA and performed in a single stage (assuming the underlying foot deformity is not severe, and, in our hands, the subtalar joint does not require arthrodesis). The talus erodes into the medial malleolus and distal tibial articular surface, resulting in a bony defect at the medial plafond. Reduction of congruent varus deformity can be difficult if the joint is rigid, or if there is fibular overgrowth preventing reduction. Our strategy in reducing these rigid deformities in a single stage is to use the anterior approach to recreate a neutral tibial plafond (90° with respect to the load-bearing axis of the tibia) by progressively removing lateral plafond bone until it matches the medial plafond defect. This may be challenging, and often involves removing posterior plafond bone as well, for the talus is often translated anteriorly. Commensurate with this, a reciprocating saw is used to progressively remove bone in the lateral gutter to allow reduction of the talus to neutral, congruent with the newly created tibial plafond (**Fig. 2A–F**). This may also require use of the reciprocating saw in the medial gutter if there are offending osteophytes present from longstanding impaction of medial bone. This method avoids the need for medial or lateral malleolar osteotomies to assist with deformity correction, and, as such, eliminates the variable of nonunion compromising the outcome of the arthroplasty.

The need for concomitant procedures (ie, closing-wedge calcaneal osteotomy, metatarsal dorsiflexion osteotomy, and modified Brostrom lateral ligament reconstruction) is assessed after the metallic components of the prosthesis are implanted (**Fig. 2G–M**). Axial fluoroscopic imaging (using a large C-arm) is useful to evaluate hindfoot alignment and determination of the necessity of closing-wedge calcaneal osteotomy (**Fig. 2H, I**). Palpation of the plantar metatarsal heads will reveal residual fixed forefoot pronation. Dorsiflexion osteotomy of the first metatarsal or dorsiflexion arthrodesis of the first tarsometatarsal joint (depending on the apex and/or magnitude of deformity) may be used to combat this problem, providing a balanced axis of load during the flat-foot and toe-off portions of the gait cycle (**Fig. 2J, K**).

Soft tissue balancing is deferred to the last step. Tibiotalar joint stability and ligament tension should be assessed with trial polyethylene at varying thickness. The appropriately sized polyethylene should tension the deltoid ligament, as this ligament often provides solid end point in varus. Although a deltoid ligament release may inevitably be necessary, we first prefer to balance the thickness of polyethylene component to match the tension of the deltoid ligament. This minimizes the occurrence of medial ankle instability (from an excessive release) and the need for a larger polyethylene component. The lateral ankle ligaments are now assessed for attenuation. In our experience, the lateral soft tissues are typically of good enough quality to perform an adequate imbrication in patients with congruent varus deformity. Although it is often less necessary to perform a lateral ligament reconstruction in congruent varus deformity, we stress the ankle with the polyethylene in place to confirm that supposition. It is mandatory that no residual varus deformity remains (**Fig. 3**). Residual varus deformity will lead to eccentric loading across the ankle prosthesis and early implant failure (**Figs. 4–7**).

Incongruent Varus Tibiotalar Deformity

The enigma surrounding incongruent varus deformity revolves around whether it can be performed in a single-stage or dual-stage operation. We are unaware of any reports on 2-stage TAA in association with preoperative varus deformity.

An incongruent deformity is more likely to be associated with deltoid ligament contracture, significant chronic lateral ankle instability, and lateral ligament attenuation (compared with congruent deformity). Therefore, we obtain stress radiographs (varus and valgus) before surgery to help quantify this laxity (**Fig. 8J**). This is a quick and cost-effective way to assess the rigidity of the tibiotalar deformity and lateral ligament complex.

Widening of the lateral ankle joint is often present and the talus is tilted into varus. Osteophytes accumulate in the lateral gutter in longstanding deformity, impeding reduction of the talus into the ankle mortise (**Fig. 8E**). The deltoid ligament and medial

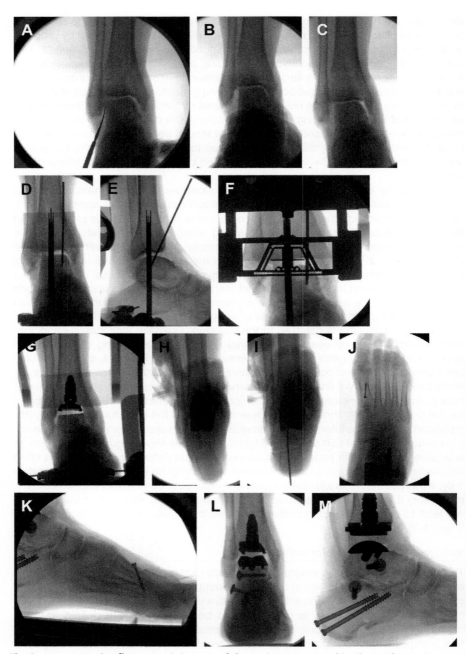

Fig. 2. Intraoperative fluoroscopic images of the patient presented in **Fig. 1**. The patient underwent a TAA with INBONE-II, closing-wedge calcaneal osteotomy, first metatarsal dorsiflexion osteotomy, and lateral ligament reconstruction. Given the reasonable quality of the lateral ligaments allowing a modified Brostrom versus a tendon transfer reconstruction, and the minimal arthritis at the subtalar joint, this procedure was performed in a single setting. The freer is being used to point out the lateral gutter exostosis that will impede

joint capsule may be contracted. The obvious goal is to correct the talus to a neutral position. Similar to a congruent deformity correction, reduction of the talus is performed through a debridement of the lateral gutter with the reciprocating saw, and again, using the saw medially to eliminate osteophytes (if present). Many surgeons begin with a deltoid ligament release, but we prefer to work on the lateral gutter first with hopes of preserving the deltoid ligament (**Fig. 9**A, B); however, it should be noted that deltoid ligament release was required in all patients (n = 23) with a varus deformity greater than 10° in an older, 2009 study.[18] At 27-month follow-up, there were no differences in American Orthopaedic Foot and Ankle Society scores and radiographic outcomes between patients with incongruent and congruent varus deformities.

It is clear that single-stage incongruent varus deformity correction is identical to single-stage congruent correction, and, as such, from this point on, we discuss 2-stage correction. We make the decision to correct a deformity through 2 separate stages based on a number of factors, including but not limited to (1) an arthritic subtalar joint that requires arthrodesis, a rigid subtalar joint with medial translation of the calcaneus upon the talus that requires arthrodesis; (2) gross lateral ligament instability with associated severe foot pathology; (3) prior attempts at cavovarus foot correction with inadequate or underpowered procedures and gross ligament instability. Please note these are not hard and fast rules, but they are general guidelines to give a surgeon pause before attempting single-stage correction. With this in mind, we evaluate some of the procedures available for correction.

Some centers prefer to address contracture of the deltoid ligament indirectly by performing a 5-mm lengthening osteotomy of the medial malleolus, obviating the need for a medial soft tissue release.[19] The investigators were able to achieve neutral postoperative alignment in 15 patients (100%) with a mean preoperative varus deformity of 14.9°; however, 2 patients developed a medial malleolus nonunion and 1 patient required revision for tibial component subsidence. There is no comparative evidence

---

reduction of the talus (*A*). The reciprocating saw was used to perform an aggressive lateral gutter debridement (*B*). Despite adequate lateral gutter debridement, the deformity was irreducible because of the medial gutter spurring and deltoid ligament contracture. Medial gutter osteophytes were debrided, lessening the tension on the deltoid ligament complex (*C*). The talus was reduced and pinned in place with a threaded wire (*D*, *E*). Erosion of the medial tibial plafond can be appreciated after placement of the cutting guide (*F*). Inevitably, more lateral distal tibia will be resected with varus deformity. The tibial stem was implanted and the threaded wire removed (*G*). The varus deformity recurs with removal of the threaded wire, indicating that further soft tissue balancing (and tensioning) was needed. This is performed after all boney work is completed, to truly appreciate the magnitude of instability present, and to allow protection of the weakest portion of the surgery (soft tissue reconstruction). Axial alignment heel radiographs reveal a congenital varus deformity of the calcaneal tuberosity (*H*). Therefore, a closing-wedge calcaneal osteotomy was performed to realign the calcaneal tuberosity in line with the long axis of the tibia (*I*). The forefoot driven component of the cavus foot was addressed through a first metatarsal dorsiflexion osteotomy (*J*, *K*). An attempt was made to tension the native lateral ligaments. However, in severe incongruent deformities, an imbrication of the lateral ligaments is typically not enough to maintain correction. Anatomic lateral ligament reconstruction was performed using a semitendinosis allograft drilled at the origin points of both the anterior talofibular and calcaneofibular ligament, and anchored with a screw/post at the insertion points of both ligaments (*L*, *M*). We prefer to downsize the polyethylene component and balance the ankle joint by performing a lateral ankle soft tissue tensioning against an intact deltoid ligament. We believe that excessive release of the deltoid ligament creates instability, which is then compensated for by using a larger sized polyethylene component.

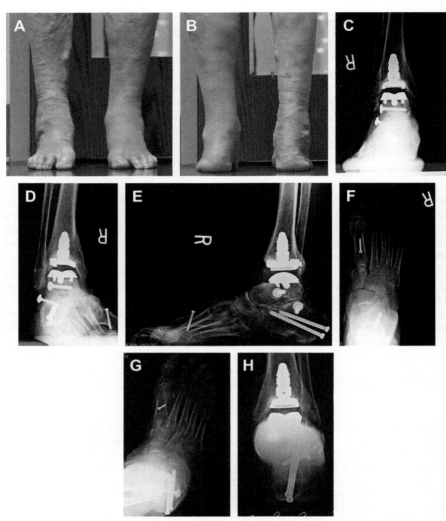

Fig. 3. Postoperative clinical photographs and radiographs 1-year after TAA of the patient presented in **Figs. 1** and **2**. There is a significant improvement in clinical alignment (*A, B*) compared with preoperative photographs (see **Fig. 1**A, B). The tibiotalar joint is congruent at 1-year follow-up, without any signs of implant failure or recurrence of the varus deformity (*C–E*). The decrease in metatarsal overlap on AP foot radiograph (*F, G*) compared with preoperative radiographs (see **Fig. 1**F, G) demonstrates de-rotation of the foot. Axial alignment radiographs demonstrate neutral alignment of the calcaneal tuberosity (*H*).

to suggest that this technique is more effective than lateral ligament reconstruction and partial medial ligament release. It is not our preference to perform such osteotomies, for bone quality of the medial malleolus is often compromised, and nonunion (and salvage thereof) is a significant concern. Regardless of the chosen method, it is mandatory that prosthetic joint stability and neutral mechanical alignment be achieved. Patient outcomes and implant survivorship are poor if there is residual malalignment (see **Figs. 4–7**).[20]

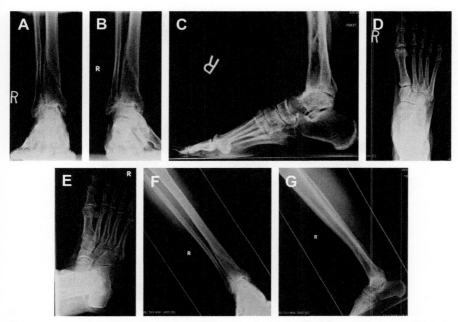

Fig. 4. Preoperative weight-bearing radiographs of a 78-year-old man with severe tibiotalar joint arthritis and a remote history of a distal tibia fracture. AP and mortise ankle radiographs demonstrate a subtle varus deformity slightly proximal to the distal tibia metadiaphysis (*A, B*). Anterior subluxation of the talus and recurvatum deformity of the distal tibia is noted on lateral radiograph (*C*). No appreciable rotational foot deformity is present on AP and oblique foot radiographs (*D, E*). The subtle distal tibia deformity is easier to identify on full-length tibia/fibula radiographs (*F, G*). Distal tibial recurvatum and varus deformity is remonstrated. The distal tibial deformity is not large enough to perform a corrective osteotomy.

After mobilization of the talus and manual correction to neutral with respect to the tibiotalar axis, we maintain this reduction using a large threaded wire traversing the tibiotalar joint, often placed laterally from the tibia into the talus. The purpose of this now static reduction is to simulate the corrected ankle joint with the prosthesis in place, so that a perfect foot alignment can be built beneath. Generally, if we are performing a 2-stage reconstruction, deformity is more severe than can be tackled with a closing-wedge Dwyer-type calcaneal osteotomy. As such, we next consider subtalar joint arthrodesis (**Fig. 9**).

Subtalar arthrodesis, when performed concurrently with TAA, may result in excessive injury to the extraosseous blood supply to the talus, which may lead to avascular necrosis and subsequent talar component subsidence.[21] Cadaveric studies demonstrate that surgical instrumentation, technique, and the type of total ankle prosthesis are all factors that result in varying degrees of vascular disruption of the arterial inflow to the talus. At least 1 major artery to the talus was violated during instrumentation and implantation regardless of the type of prosthesis (INBONE-II, Scandinavian Total Ankle Replacement [STAR], Salto Talaris, and Trabecular Metal Total Ankle).[21] We dispute these findings, as the in vivo incidence of talar avascular necrosis (AVN) does not appear to correlate with the high rates of vascular injury reported in this particular cadaveric study.[22] Regardless, there is concern that there is greater disruption to

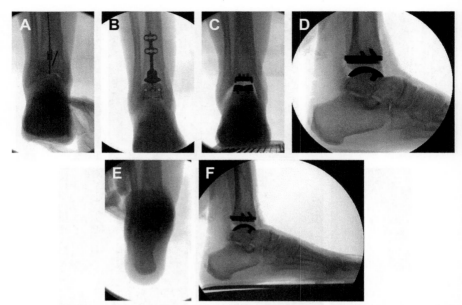

Fig. 5. The patient (presented in **Fig. 4**) underwent an INFINITY TAA with CT-guided patient specific instrumentation. The CT protocol references proximal anatomic landmarks to determine the appropriate mechanical alignment, rotation, and level of bone resection. CT-guided protocols can be advantageous in cases with mild extra-articular deformity, as in this particular case, when the mechanical axis of the tibia deviates from its anatomic axis. There are multiple fluoroscopic "check points" to ensure that the distal tibia and talar bone resections are performed perpendicular to the mechanical axis of the tibia (*A, B*). Final intraoperative radiographs demonstrate a low-profile total ankle prosthesis in appropriate alignment (*C, D*). Intraoperative axial alignment radiographs demonstrate a subtle congenital varus deformity of the calcaneal tuberosity (*E*), while simulated weight-bearing radiographs reveal a slight increase in calcaneal pitch and a very mild cavovarus deformity (*F*). No concomitant procedures were performed at the time of TAA.

the talar blood supply when TAA and subtalar arthrodesis are performed at the same time. As such, if the patient requires a subtalar arthrodesis, we recommend performing this as a 2-stage procedure. It is acceptable to perform a talonavicular and/or calcaneocuboid joint arthrodesis at the time of TAA, as there is less concern for injury to the talar blood supply.

The technique we prefer for subtalar joint arthrodesis in cavovarus deformity involves a flat-cut, closing-wedge method using a macrosagittal saw. Despite the presence of the fibula, access is possible to the entire posterior facet with this saw. In fact, it is somewhat easier in cavovarus, as the fibula is often translated posteriorly. The residual cartilage is denuded using an AO chisel. Distraction is critical within the subtalar joint. We remove both the anterior and middle facet continuity using a high-speed burr under iced irrigation.[23] This is a critical step to allow compression of the posterior facet of the subtalar joint, and may even require removal of bone at the medial side of the anterior neck of the calcaneus and a portion of the lateral part of the talar head (we spend significant time here making certain there are no distracting elements at this portion of the foot to allow deformity correction at the posterior facet by providing a recess for the talar head). Final preparation of the posterior facet is now performed

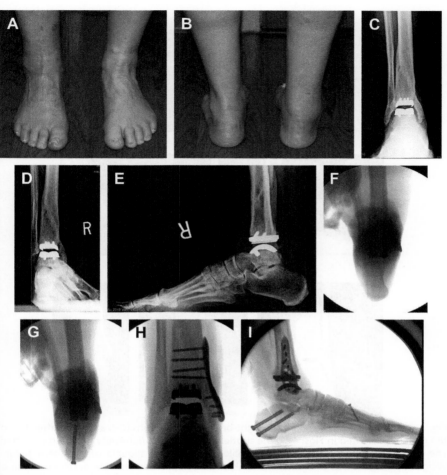

Fig. 6. Clinical photographs 4 months after TAA reveal a subtle, persistent cavovarus deformity of the right foot (*A, B*). This foot deformity, along with the subtle distal tibia varus malunion, was enough to shift the weight-bearing vector medially, resulting in a stress fracture of the medial malleolus (*C–E*). Despite the fracture, the implant remained stable. The patient underwent a second procedure to correct the residual cavovarus deformity and plate the medial malleolus fracture. Intraoperative axial alignment radiographs demonstrate a congenital varus deformity of the calcaneal tuberosity (*F*), which was corrected with a lateral closing-wedge calcaneal osteotomy (*G*). An anatomically contoured distal tibial plate was used to rigidly fixate the medial malleolus fracture (*H*) and a first metatarsal dorsiflexion osteotomy was performed to correct the subtle forefoot pronation (*I*).

with a flat cut at both the talar and calcaneal portions of the subtalar joint. Bone preservation is critical, and thus the macrosagittal blade is used to feather the bone to fit perfectly in contact, maximizing surface area, and providing a stable construct for perpendicular compression screw fixation. In cavovarus, we usually perform these cuts through a closing-wedge approach, the apex being the medial border of the posterior facet. We do not begin with a large wedge; instead, we resect a minimal wedge of subchondral bone, then progressively check axial fluoroscopic images with a large

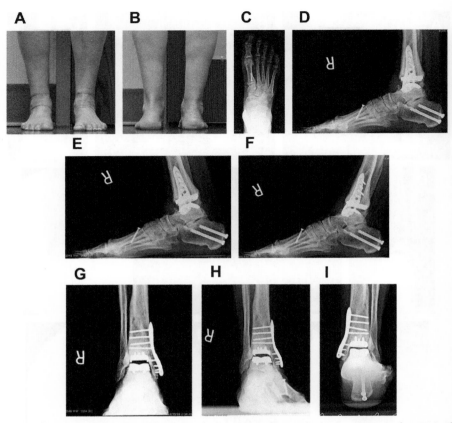

Fig. 7. Photographs (*A, B*) and final weight-bearing radiographs (*C–I*) at 3 years after TAA of the patient presented in **Figs. 4–6**. The subtle cavovarus foot deformity has been corrected. The medial malleolus fracture is well healed without any sequela of prosthesis failure. Weight-bearing flexion and extension ankle radiographs demonstrate excellent range of motion and well-functioning implant.

C-arm until the varus deformity of the hindfoot is reduced to neutral. We monitor the congruence between the talus and calcaneus laterally, to ensure we have corrected the lateral overhang of the talus commonly seen at the subtalar joint in cavovarus. Finally, preserving the declination angle of the posterior facet ensures the talus maintains the corrected Meary angle without dorsiflexion or plantarflexion. In our opinion, this is a true reconstruction, and significant time should be spent to ensure it is perfect.

At this point, we assess for residual lateral column overload. Simulated weight-bearing lateral fluoroscopic images will dictate whether the fifth ray is off-loaded sufficiently. In patients with a preserved talonavicular joint, with good cartilage, we prefer to correct this overload through the calcaneocuboid joint. The calcaneocuboid joint is distracted, allowing direct visualization of its saddle-shaped architecture. Commonly, an adduction deformity is present in cavovarus, requiring the use of a microsagittal saw to flat cut the calcaneocuboid joint in anticipation of creating a closing-wedge osteotomy through this joint. An added benefit of the flat cuts is the increased ability to vertically translate the cuboid at the fusion site, offloading the lateral column through distal elevation. One can aggressively elevate the lateral column through

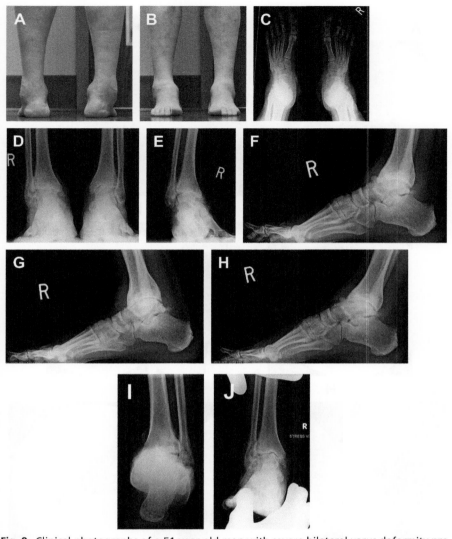

Fig. 8. Clinical photographs of a 51-year-old man with severe bilateral varus deformity present at the tibiotalar joint (*A, B*). The patient underwent a right 2-stage cavovarus correction. The weight-bearing AP foot radiograph demonstrates a severe rotational foot deformity with significant overlap of the metatarsals (*C*). Ankle radiographs demonstrate a severe bilateral incongruent varus deformity with erosion of the medial tibial plafond and lateral gutter osteophyte formation (*D–F*). The right ankle deformity is more severe, with preoperative ultrasound documenting absence of lateral ligament complex. Flexion and extension radiographs of the ankle demonstrate limited functional range of motion (*G, H*). The axial heel alignment radiograph demonstrates a varus position of the calcaneal tuberosity (*I*). Although there does appear to be a slight congenital varus deformity of the calcaneal tuberosity, the magnitude of the hindfoot varus deformity cannot fully be appreciated without a preoperative weight-bearing CT and intraoperative radiographs with the tibiotalar joint corrected to neutral (as a portion of the hindfoot deformity is driven by the varus incongruence at the tibiotalar joint). Reverse stress radiographs further reveal the sulcus in the medial tibial plafond, and the inability to reduce the ankle joint to neutral (with both lateral blocking osteophytes and medial deltoid tension) (*J*).

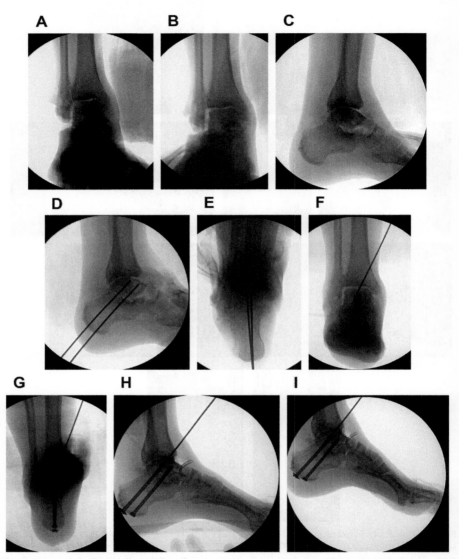

Fig. 9. Intraoperative radiographs of a cavovarus reconstruction through a closing-wedge subtalar joint arthrodesis, first metatarsal dorsiflexion osteotomy, lateral ligament reconstruction, and tibiotalar joint cement spacer (patient presented in **Fig. 8**). The sinus tarsi approach is used to perform the subtalar joint arthrodesis. The lateral gutter is accessible through this incision as well. Adequate lateral gutter debridement must be performed to reduce the talus. Reverse stress radiographs demonstrate that the talus is reducible to neutral after debridement of the lateral gutter (A–C). We perform an aggressive lateral gutter debridement during the first stage, so that the lateral ligament reconstruction is not inadvertently injured during the second stage. To minimize the risk of regrowth of lateral bone into the gutter between stages, we liberally apply bone wax to the cut surfaces. We perform a closing-wedge subtalar joint arthrodesis by making flat cuts with a macrosagittal saw. The flat cut increases bony apposition, stability, and congruency (and allows increasing corrective power) for successful subtalar joint arthrodesis (D). It is important to assess axial

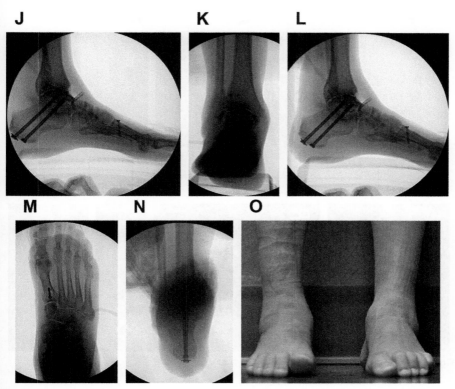

Fig. 9. (*continued*).

heel alignment after placing guide wires (*E*). If there is residual malalignment (despite correction through the subtalar joint), then a concomitant calcaneal osteotomy can be performed. We felt that an isolated subtalar joint arthrodesis was sufficient; therefore, the calcaneal osteotomy was deferred in this particular case (although we recognize that if there is residual varus, we can address that more simply with a closing-wedge calcaneal osteotomy at the second stage). The tibiotalar joint was corrected to neutral and reduction was held with a large treaded wire (*F*). The bone tunnel in the distal fibula from the lateral ligament reconstruction is noted on AP ankle radiographs. Heel alignment can change after correction of the talus to neutral; therefore, it is important to obtain axial heel alignment radiographs at multiple points throughout the surgery to reconfirm that the heel is indeed in a neutral position and aligned with the anatomic axis of tibia (with the second toe rotated in *line* with the center of the tibia) (*G*). The simulated lateral weight-bearing radiograph demonstrates a forefoot-driven cavus deformity (*H*), which was corrected with a first metatarsal dorsiflexion osteotomy (*I, J*). Cement was injected into the ankle joint before removal of the threaded wire (*K*), which serves to protect the lateral ligament reconstruction by maintaining tibiotalar joint congruency and removing tension off the ligament reconstruction. Final intraoperative radiographs demonstrate correction of the ankle and foot deformity (*K–N*). At 13 weeks after the first stage, clinical photographs (*O, P*) and weight-bearing radiographs (*Q–U*) demonstrate almost complete correction of the deformity. There is mild residual varus deformity still present at the tibiotalar joint (*R*). However, this will easily be corrected with an aggressive medial gutter debridement, conservative deltoid ligament release, and an appropriately sized polyethylene component at the time of TAA.

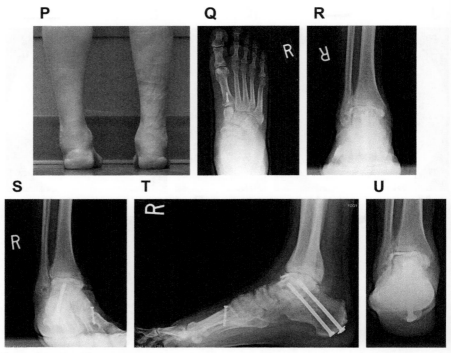

Fig. 9. (*continued*).

this method, using the hemispherical talonavicular joint as a fulcrum to rotate about. Fixation is easily done at this location with a compression plate, and, against flat surfaces of bone apposition, union rates are high.

As with congruent deformities, the next step in reconstruction involves addressing the pronation of the first ray. The need for this procedure is easily detected clinically, by placing one's thumb beneath the first or fifth metatarsal (depending on right or left foot, respectively) and the opposite hand thumb on the fifth or first metatarsal. Pressing superiorly will confirm a plantarflexed first ray. This rotational component must be addressed. We assess the apex of this deformity by sagittal plane imaging, and most often the apex presents at the first metatarsocuneiform joint. If there is not such a "humpback" deformity, the closing-wedge osteotomy is done at the base of the first ray, made oblique to facilitate screw fixation (see **Fig. 9**H–J).

The lateral ligament complex is the next component to be addressed. We have already addressed the modified Brostrom procedure, and if the ligaments are of good quality, that procedure is appropriate. More often than not, however, with deformities severe enough to be considered for 2-stage reconstruction, imbrication of the lateral ligaments is insufficient. In addition, one advantage of the sinus tarsi approach for subtalar arthrodesis is direct access to the lateral gutter of the ankle joint. This ensures excellent lateral gutter debridement and eradication of any potential impinging osteophytes that may later compromise TAA. The time to perform aggressive gutter debridement is now, rather than at the time of the TAA, when secondary ligament violation during such a debridement may compromise all of the index work that was performed during the first stage. We apply bone wax over exposed bony surfaces to minimize the risk of heterotopic ossification and regrowth to keep the gutter patent for the arthroplasty.

Assuming poor-quality lateral ligament tissue, we choose to perform an anatomic lateral ligament reconstruction using semitendinosus allograft tendon. The skin incision used for the subtalar fusion is acceptable, although it is extended curvilinear inferior and posterior to the fibula. One must identify and protect the sural nerve, as longstanding neuralgia will compromise the entire reconstructive effort. The insertion of the anterior talofibular ligament (ATFL) is identified at the junction of the talar body and neck. A Beath needle is directed into the talar body (inferior and posterior trajectory). A second Beath needle is placed at the insertion of the calcaneofibular ligament, directed inferior and medial, to exit the medial skin avoiding the tibial nerve and artery. An acorn reamer 7.5 mm in diameter is drilled to a depth of 25 mm in the talus, and 30 mm in the calcaneus, over each Beath needle. Final tunnel preparation is done by drilling 4.0-mm bone tunnels at a 90/90 angle through the origins of the ATFL and calcaneofibular ligament, meeting in the central distal fibula. We do not violate the posterior cortex of the fibula, as this increases the chance of a distal fibula fracture.

The allograft tendon is tubularized, and one end of this tendon has a Krakow weave stitch placed through it with permanent suture. This limb is passed into the talar tunnel after putting this suture through the eyelet of the Beath needle and pulling the Beath needle through medially. Tension is applied, and a 7 × 23- mm interference screw is placed into the talar tunnel, securing the graft. The graft is then passed through the 90/90 bone tunnel in the fibula with a Hewson passer. If diameter of the tunnel hole is too small, it is expanded with a curved curette. Maximum tension is again placed on this allograft, and the allograft is secured in the ATFL drill hole of the fibula with a 4.5-mm interference screw. The distance between the inferior fibula drill hole and the calcaneal drill hole is measured, and this measurement is added to the tunnel depth measurement of 25 mm (to allow some additional tension to be placed on the graft). The graft is then cut at this length (the graft length is measured from the inferior tip of the fibula), and a Krackow weave performed. This suture end is then placed through the eyelet of the Beath needle, and the Beath needle is pulled through the hindfoot medially. One must remember to ensure the graft is traveling deep to the peroneal tendons to avoid entrapment before fixation. The sutures are pulled tightly from where they exit the medial hindfoot, and with this tension, the graft is fixed at the calcaneal tunnel with an additional 7 × 23- mm interference screw. Any additional available soft tissue (or former ligament) can complement this repair by anchoring it to the periosteum of the fibula.

With this stout repair completed, one last step is necessary. To keep tension off the graft repair, and maintain neutral alignment, we now inject cement into the medial portion of the tibiotalar joint. If cartilage is present at that site, we burr this off to create an exposed subchondral surface that will assist with the cement staying in place during weight bearing. Once the cement hardens, the threaded pin initially placed traversing the tibiotalar joint is removed. The cement provides a dual benefit. It takes the tension off of the ligament repair laterally by maintaining the parallel nature of the corrected tibiotalar joint, and it allows standing and earlier weight bearing (assuming fusions are progressing) to minimize disuse osteopenia in advance of the TAA.

The compression wrap protocol is immediately instituted and maintained for the first 2.5 weeks.[13,24] The extremity may then be casted for 4 additional weeks, followed by cast removal and standing weight bearing assuming CT scan confirmation of progressive arthrodesis. Before the second stage (traditionally at 13–14 weeks following the first stage), the compression wrap protocol is instituted again 1 week before to minimize extremity edema at the time of the second surgery.

The second stage may be performed with the TAA of choice (**Figs. 10** and **11**). The interposed cement is traditionally left in place, and removed along with the saw cuts for the chosen prosthesis. One must be careful to ensure the bone is of good quality

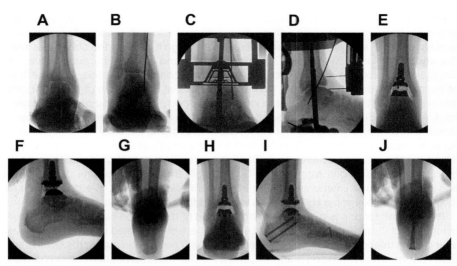

Fig. 10. Intraoperative radiographs of the second-stage TAA with a stemmed tibial implant 13 weeks after the index operation (patient presented in **Figs. 8** and **9**). The tibiotalar joint remained congruent after removal of the cement (*A*). The reduction is maintained with a threaded guide wire, which is placed out of the way of the bone resection guide (*B-D*). All the bone cuts must be started with the threaded guide wire in place. However, if the threaded guide wire interferes with any of the bone cuts, it can later be removed to finish the bone cuts after the cutting block guide is pinned in position. The final tibial component has been implanted (*E, F*). The ankle is congruent with the trial polyethylene and talar components in place. However, sometimes we revise the talar bone cut, free hand, with a macrosagittal saw when necessary. Although the calcaneal tuberosity is aligned with the long axis of the tibia, there is still a slight congenital varus of the tuberosity, which was corrected through a closing-wedge calcaneal osteotomy (*G*). Final intraoperative radiographs demonstrate appropriately aligned total ankle prosthesis with complete elimination of the varus deformity (*H–J*).

on this second surgery, and, if not, ensure the prosthesis is robust enough to cover any defects. Also in the second stage, if the surgeon wishes to add additional minor procedures to compensate for any residual varus (ie, a closing-wedge Dwyer-type calcaneal osteotomy), they may be performed without compromising early motion of the ankle joint prosthesis.

The goal of the second stage is early aggressive ankle motion. We have found that if we immobilize the ankle prosthesis following implantation, the ankle invariably becomes stiffer. Early motion is instituted, along with the compression wrap protocol to both minimize the risk of secondary incision complications, and minimize the edema in the extremity, which would compromise motion. We restrict standing or weight bearing in these complex staged reconstructions for 6 weeks to facilitate ingrowth of the prosthesis. There is no real benefit to earlier weight bearing if one is already achieving good motion through early physical therapy protocols.

When neutral alignment is achieved, functional outcomes are found to be similar regardless of the severity of preoperative deformity.[25] Approximately 70% of patients with severe preoperative varus deformity (25.7°) compared with only 35% of patients with mild varus deformity (4.9°) required ancillary procedures at the time of TAA.[18] Ancillary procedures performed included lateral ankle ligament repair, percutaneous Achilles tendon lengthening, supramalleolar osteotomy, medial malleolar sliding osteotomy, peroneal tendon transfer, lateral calcaneal closing-wedge osteotomy,

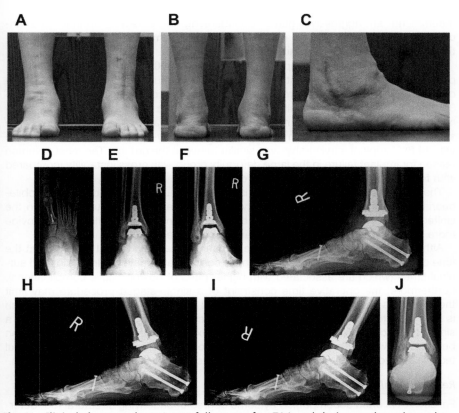

Fig. 11. Clinical photographs at 1-year follow-up after TAA and closing-wedge calcaneal osteotomy on the right side (*A, B*). The patient underwent a varus correction, single-stage TAA on the left side. There is significant improvement in alignment compared with preoperative clinical photographs (see **Fig. 8**A, B). We minimize the risk of incisional wound complications through a compression wrap protocol after surgery (and before surgery). Despite the close proximity of the lateral hindfoot incisions, we believe that a perfect bony correction must not be compromised with concern of the small lateral skin bridge (*C*). The rotational foot deformity, although mostly driven by the ankle and hindfoot varus, is significantly improved (*D*) compared with preoperative foot radiographs (see **Fig. 8**C). Final weight-bearing ankle radiographs demonstrate a stable ankle prosthesis with complete correction of the incongruent varus tibiotalar and cavovarus foot deformities and excellent range of motion not possible with a tibiotalocalcaneal joint arthrodesis (*E–J*).

dorsiflexion osteotomy of the first metatarsal, and subtalar arthrodesis. There were no differences in clinical outcomes, postoperative pain, or implant survivorship at an average of 34.2-month follow-up.

Trajkovski and colleagues[25] reported similar findings. Twenty-nine patients (81%) with varus deformity, compared with 17 patients (47%) with neutral alignment, required ancillary procedures at the time of total ankle replacement. Patients with a preoperative varus deformity were twice as likely to undergo a second surgery compared with patients with neutral alignment. Five patients in the varus group required repeat surgery because of lateral gutter impingement and persistent pain. Despite the higher rate of subsequent surgeries performed in the varus cohort, there was no difference in clinical outcome or implant survivorship between the groups. We recommend an aggressive gutter debridement, as tibiotalar arthritis is a tri-compartmental disease, and inadequate gutter debridement can result in postoperative stiffness, pain, and subsequent failure.

Hobson and colleagues[26] reported on more than 100 consecutive total ankle replacements with the STAR prosthesis. Patients were grouped according to the degree of preoperative tibiotalar deformity (less than 10° of coronal plane deformity vs 11°–30° of deformity). Varus deformity was significantly more prevalent than valgus deformity. Postoperative range of motion, complications, and patient outcomes were similar across the groups. At an average of 4-year follow-up, the overall rate of failure was 14.6%. Implant survivorship was similar between the groups. The most common reason for implant failure in the large deformity group was gross instability (compared with fracture in the group with minimal deformity).

The generalizability of these studies is limited because they are based on mobile-bearing implants, including the Mobility and Hintegra, which are unavailable in the United States. We believe that fixed-bearing implants are beneficial and provide more stability when larger deformities are being addressed.

Although some investigators are able to achieve plantigrade foot alignment at the time of TAA, it is a technically demanding procedure and may require prolonged surgical times (which are associated with higher rates of postoperative complications). Furthermore, the operative time constraint of a single-staged procedure may limit the surgeon's capacity to adequately correct all aspects of the foot deformity, which is necessary to achieve an excellent, long-term clinical outcome. We advise against a single-stage correction for surgeons with less experience. Successful outcomes can be achieved with 2-staged varus correction. Thoughtful surgical planning and careful technical execution minimizes the risk of a catastrophic failure for the next surgeon.

Revision Total Ankle Arthroplasty

Failed TAA is often accompanied by some degree of underlying structural foot deformity. Residual foot malalignment is a major cause of early prosthesis failure following TAA. Persistent cavovarus deformity pushes the weight-bearing axis medial, resulting in an eccentric load through the tibiotalar joint and eventual varus failure of the metal prosthesis. We frequently find that the foot deformity was unrecognized, ignored, or poorly corrected at the time of the primary TAA. In our experience, the bony deficits associated with severe implant subsidence and residual structural foot deformity often mandates 2-stage correction.

After the surgeon commits to a 2-stage correction, the severity of the residual foot deformity is the major determinant as to whether an extra-articular reconstruction can be attempted or a hindfoot arthrodesis is required. We believe that a hindfoot arthrodesis should be considered (over a second attempt extra-articular cavovarus reconstruction) in the following situations: hindfoot arthritis, AVN of the talus, talar component subsidence with bone loss, and severe cavovarus deformity. Hindfoot arthrodesis is a reliable way to correct the underlying deformity while maintaining adequate bone stock for a revision TAA.

If there is only mild residual foot deformity, then a second attempt at an extra-articular correction may be attempted. Axial heel alignment radiographs are useful to determine the need for revision calcaneal osteotomy. The surgeon should consider a closing-wedge calcaneal osteotomy if congenital varus of the calcaneus is present. The calcaneal tuberosity should be aligned with the axis of the tibia on intraoperative axial heel alignment radiographs. Lateral translation of the calcaneal osteotomy creates an increased risk of tibial neuralgia after surgery, which can be debilitating.[27,28] The cavus deformity can be corrected through a first metatarsal dorsiflexion osteotomy or a dorsal midfoot closing-wedge osteotomy and arthrodesis (performed at the apex of deformity). We choose to perform the latter when there is a large cavus deformity and structural bony support is needed for the revision prosthesis. The INVIS-ION (Wright Medical, Memphis, TN) prosthesis achieves bony fixation through a talar baseplate that can be extended distal to maximize surface contact area with the healthy cortical bone of the talar neck or dorsal navicular. It has been our experience that the anterior extent of the talar baseplate must reside on quality cortical bone and it is sometimes necessary to perform a talonavicular arthrodesis to achieve appropriate structural support for the metal prosthesis. In such cases, the cavovarus deformity should be corrected through a realignment arthrodesis at the talonavicular joint. After structural realignment is performed, the soft tissues must be balanced. However, we typically defer soft tissue balancing until the second stage.

The objective of the first surgery is to careful removal of the prosthesis (to minimize bone loss) and concurrent correction of any residual structural foot malalignment. Typically, there is very little bone ingrowth present and the implants are grossly unstable. Osteotomes can be used to lever the metal components free. If the prosthesis is fixed, then a reciprocating saw can be used at the implant–bone interface to free the component while minimizing bone loss. After the prosthesis is removed, necrotic bone is debrided with a curette and power burr. Following debridement, a Steinman pin is placed through the calcaneal tuberosity. The pin is used to distract the ankle joint and hold the talus in a neutral position while antibiotic cement is injected into the joint using a 60-mL syringe. After the cement hardens, we reassess the foot for residual structural deformity. Correction of the foot deformity is performed as detailed previously. We do not perform any soft tissue procedures during the first stage, as ligament tension can change after final implantation of the prosthesis at the time of the second-stage procedure. The caveat to this rule is if no ligaments are present laterally, and, in that case, we perform the semitendinosis allograft procedure mentioned previously.

The second stage is performed 13 to 14 weeks after the index surgery, allowing adequate time for the realignment osteotomies/arthrodesis to heal and soft tissue swelling to mitigate. We obtain a weight-bearing CT 3 months after the initial surgery to confirm successful union. We recommend using a stemmed tibial implant for revision TAA, particularly when prosthesis failure occurred secondary to preexisting coronal malalignment.

The antibiotic cement is removed from the tibiotalar joint in a piecemeal fashion, which is facilitated by dividing the cement into quadrants using a reciprocating saw and osteotomes. We remove any remaining necrotic bone and tissue using the power burr with iced irrigation.

In the presence of significant central talar cavitary defects following catastrophic failure, we have modified our cement techniques traditionally used beneath the prosthesis. First, we place the trial components. Guide wires from the cannulated screw set are placed in a retrograde fashion from the plantar aspect of the calcaneus and into the cavitary defect of the talus. The number of guide wires used depends on the extent of talar bone loss. The goal is for the guide wires to buttress the talar component from subsiding into the cavitary defect, as such, the guide wires must be the perfect length to achieve this effect. If the guide wires are too short, then the talar component will subside. Similarly, if the guide wires are too long, the metal talar component will tilt creating incongruence at the joint. We use intraoperative fluoroscopy to confirm appropriate guide wire length. 4.0-mm fully threaded cannulated screws are advanced in a retrograde fashion over top the guide wires. At times, it may be necessary to washers to "fine-tune" final length of the screw. At this time, cement is mixed and placed in a 60-mL syringe. If the cavitary talar defect is uncontained, we use osteotomes in the gutter to contain the cement as it in carefully injected into the defect. Pressurized injection of the cement into the defect is typically enough to fill all areas of bony void; however, fluoroscopy is useful to confirm that the cement reaches the posterior aspect of the cavitary defect. We use a freer to mold the cement as is hardens. The osteotomes are left in place until the cement is completely hardened. We have found that our "rebar" technique provides a stable platform for the metal talar prosthesis.

After final implantation of the ankle prosthesis, the structural anatomy of the foot is reassessed for the need to perform additional realignment. We are very meticulous to obtain high-quality intraoperative simulated weight-bearing radiographs to ensure that there is no residual cavovarus deformity. We recommend liberal use of fluoroscopy and a flat plate to help assist with this process. Occasionally, it is necessary to achieve additional correction by removing the hardware and revising the osteotomy (performed during the first stage). The soft tissues are balanced last.

There is paucity in literature on 2-stage varus correction. In fact, we are unaware of any studies that report on the outcomes following 2-stage varus correction. Successful outcomes have been reported with cavovarus correction at the time of TAA (single-stage).[12,18,25,26,29] As long as neutral mechanical alignment and prosthetic joint stability are achieved during the operation, whether performed as a single-stage or 2-stage procedure, good outcomes can be expected. In our experience, there are only a few absolute indications for a 2-stage varus correction: concomitant lower extremity deformity that requires surgical realignment, failed TAA, and subtalar arthrodesis. However, acceptable short-term results have been reported following TAA and concomitant subtalar arthrodesis in patients with greater than 20° of varus deformity.[29]

The senior author (SLH) has spent most of his career undertaking severe foot and ankle deformities and has learned that excellent outcomes are achievable if the principles of reconstruction and arthroplasty are respected. There is no substitution for meticulous preoperative planning and intraoperative technical execution.

REFERENCES

1. Little BS, Wixson RL, Stulberg SD. Total hip arthroplasty with the porous-coated anatomic hip prosthesis. J Arthroplasty 2006;21(3):338–43.

2. Eskelinen A, Remes V, Helenius I, et al. Uncemented total hip arthroplasty for primary osteoarthritis in young patients: a mid-to long-term follow-up study from the Finnish Arthroplasty Register. Acta Orthop 2006;77(1):57–70.

3. Kim YH, Kim JS, Cho SH. Primary total hip arthroplasty with a cementless porous-coated anatomic total hip prosthesis: 10- to 12-year results of prospective and consecutive series. J Arthroplasty 1999;14(5):538–48. Available at: http://www.ncbi.nlm.nih.gov/pubmed/10475551. Accessed January 31, 2019.

4. Kim Y-H. Long-term results of the cementless porous-coated anatomic total hip prosthesis. J Bone Joint Surg Br 2005;87-B(5):623–7.

5. Stinchfield FE, Eftekhar N. THE CLASSIC: dislocation and instability complicating low friction arthroplasty of the hip joint. Clin Orthop Relat Res 2006;447:4–8.

6. Dobzyniak M, Fehring TK, Odum S. Early failure in total hip arthroplasty. Clin Orthop Relat Res 2006;447:76–8.

7. Clohisy JC, Calvert G, Tull F, et al. Reasons for revision hip surgery: a retrospective review. Clin Orthop Relat Res 2004;429:188–92. Available at: http://www.ncbi.nlm.nih.gov/pubmed/15577486. Accessed January 31, 2019.

8. Le DH, Goodman SB, Maloney WJ, et al. Current modes of failure in TKA: infection, instability, and stiffness predominate. Clin Orthop Relat Res 2014;472(7): 2197–200.

9. Liau JJ, Cheng CK, Huang CH, et al. The effect of malalignment on stresses in polyethylene component of total knee prostheses–a finite element analysis. Clin Biomech (Bristol, Avon) 2002;17(2):140–6. Available at: http://www.ncbi.nlm.nih. gov/pubmed/11832264. Accessed January 31, 2019.

10. Reddy SC, Mann JA, Mann RA, et al. Correction of moderate to severe coronal plane deformity with the STAR™ ankle prosthesis. Foot Ankle Int 2011;32(7): 659–64.

11. Haskell A, Mann RA. Ankle arthroplasty with preoperative coronal plane deformity: short-term results. Clin Orthop Relat Res 2004;424:98–103. Available at: http://www.ncbi.nlm.nih.gov/pubmed/15241149. Accessed January 31, 2019.

12. Queen RM, Adams SB, Viens NA, et al. Differences in outcomes following total ankle replacement in patients with neutral alignment compared with tibiotalar joint malalignment. J Bone Joint Surg Am 2013;95(21):1927–34.

13. Schipper ON, Hsu AR, Haddad SL. Reduction in wound complications after total ankle arthroplasty using a compression wrap protocol. Foot Ankle Int 2015; 36(12):1448–54.

14. Hsu AR, Haddad SL. Early clinical and radiographic outcomes of intramedullary-fixation total ankle arthroplasty. J Bone Joint Surg Am 2015;97(3):194–200.

15. Tarr RR, Resnick CT, Wagner KS, et al. Changes in tibiotalar joint contact areas following experimentally induced tibial angular deformities. Clin Orthop Relat Res 1985;199:72–80. Available at: http://www.ncbi.nlm.nih.gov/pubmed/ 4042499. Accessed January 8, 2019.

16. Steginsky B, Riley A, Lucas DE, et al. Patient-reported outcomes and return to activity after peroneus brevis repair. Foot Ankle Int 2016;37(2):178–85.

17. Saltzman CL, El-Khoury GY. The hindfoot alignment view. Foot Ankle Int 1995; 16(9):572–6.

18. Kim BS, Choi WJ, Kim YS, et al. Total ankle replacement in moderate to severe varus deformity of the ankle. J Bone Joint Surg Br 2009;91(9):1183–90.

19. Doets HC, van der Plaat LW, Klein J-P. Medial malleolar osteotomy for the correction of varus deformity during total ankle arthroplasty: results in 15 ankles. Foot Ankle Int 2008;29(2):171–7.

20. Doets HC, Brand R, Nelissen RGHH. Total ankle arthroplasty in inflammatory joint disease with use of two mobile-bearing designs. J Bone Joint Surg Am 2006; 88(6):1272–84.

21. Tennant JN, Rungprai C, Pizzimenti MA, et al. Risks to the blood supply of the talus with four methods of total ankle arthroplasty. J Bone Joint Surg Am 2014; 96(5):395–402.

22. Hsu AR, Haddad SL. Risks to the blood supply of the talus with four methods of total ankle arthroplasty. No two arthritic ankles are the same: commentary on an article by Joshua N. Tennant, MD, MPH, et al. J Bone Joint Surg Am 2014;96(5): 395–402.

23. Haddad SL, Hsu AR, Templin CR, et al. Effects of continuous irrigation during burring on thermal necrosis and fusion strength in a rabbit arthrodesis model. Foot Ankle Int 2014;35(8):796–801.

24. Hsu AR, Franceschina D, Haddad SL. A novel method of postoperative wound care following total ankle arthroplasty. Foot Ankle Int 2014;35(7):719–24.

25. Trajkovski T, Pinsker E, Cadden A, et al. Outcomes of ankle arthroplasty with pre-operative coronal-plane varus deformity of 10° or greater. J Bone Joint Surg Am 2013;95(15):1382–8.

26. Hobson SA, Karantana A, Dhar S. Total ankle replacement in patients with significant pre-operative deformity of the hindfoot. J Bone Joint Surg Br 2009;91(4): 481–6.

27. VanValkenburg S, Hsu RY, Palmer DS, et al. Neurologic deficit associated with lateralizing calcaneal osteotomy for cavovarus foot correction. Foot Ankle Int 2016; 37(10):1106–12.

28. Krause FG, Pohl MJ, Penner MJ, et al. Tibial nerve palsy associated with lateralizing calcaneal osteotomy: case reviews and technical tip. Foot Ankle Int 2009; 30(3):258–61.

29. Sung K-S, Ahn J, Lee K-H, et al. Short-term results of total ankle arthroplasty for end-stage ankle arthritis with severe varus deformity. Foot Ankle Int 2014;35(3): 225–31.

Total Replacement of Varus Ankle

Three-Component Prosthesis Design

Beat Hintermann, MD*, Roxa Ruiz, MD

KEYWORDS

- Ankle osteoarthritis • Total ankle replacement • Varus deformity • Varus instability
- 3-component ankle prosthesis

KEY POINTS

- In most cases, a varus, misaligned, unstable ankle needs additional surgeries after a 3-component total ankle replacement to become balanced.
- Balancing the ankle using osteotomies above, at, and below the ankle in combination with soft tissue releases (medial side) and reconstruction (lateral side) is crucial for patient treatment.
- Radiographic assessment includes bilateral, weight-bearing anteroposterior and lateral views of the foot and ankle and hindfoot alignment view. Weight-bearing computed tomography can be helpful in identifying and quantifying degenerative changes, malposition, and deformities of the hindfoot.
- Long-term success highly depends on the extent to which the surgeon was able to balance the ankle.

INTRODUCTION

In the past few decades, total ankle replacement (TAR) has become an increasingly recommended and accepted treatment in patients with end-stage ankle osteoarthritis (OA).[1–12] However, controversy still exists about the appropriate indications for TAR,[13–17] specifically in ankles with coronal plane deformities. These concerns are particularly true for patients with a varus deformity, where the talus has tilted into varus within the ankle mortise due to a medial soft tissue contracture and lateral soft tissue incompetence. While standing, the center of force transmission is medialized. The forces within the joint are amplified by activation of the triceps surae, and the Achilles tendon may become an invertor,[13] thereby acting as an additional deforming force on the hindfoot.

The authors have nothing to disclose.
Clinic of Orthopaedic Surgery, Kantonsspital Baselland, Rheinstrasse 26, Liestal CH-4410, Switzerland
* Corresponding author.
E-mail address: beat.hintermann@ksbl.ch

Theoretically, the malalignment can be addressed intraoperatively with correcting cuts, but there are obvious limitations. Additional measures are necessary to obtain a balanced ankle, namely osteotomies with the specific aims of (1) realigning the hindfoot, (2) transferring the ankle joint under the weight-bearing axis, and (3) normalizing the direction of the force vector of the triceps surae.[18–20] These measures are particularly crucial when implanting a 3-component total ankle system, where the second interface of the prosthesis allows the polyethylene insert to freely translate and rotate on the flat surface of the tibial component.[21] Although not explicitly proved, the long-term success of TAR seems to largely depend on the extent to which the surgeon is able to balance the ankle joint complex.[3,22]

Indications and Contraindications for Total Ankle Replacement

TAR has become a widely accepted treatment option in patients with end-stage ankle OA. However, in varus malaligned and/or varus unstable ankles, the success of TAR depends on how well the surgeon is able to balance and stabilize the ankle. This is particularly true when using a 3-component total ankle system, which is able to adapt its axis of rotation to the patient's osteoarthritic ankle; however, it does not provide intrinsic stability to the ankle.[23,24]

The relative contraindications include a significantly reduced ankle dorsiflexion power due to neurologic disorders where active dorsiflexion may be weakened or unable to be improved postoperatively.[13] Extensive scars around the ankle and atrophy of the periarticular soft tissue mantle is another relative contraindication for TAR.[25] The absolute contraindications for TAR include acute or chronic infections with or without osteomyelitis, nonmanageable hindfoot malalignment and/or instability, and neuromuscular disorders with or without neuroarthropathy.[13,24,26,27]

Preoperative Planning

Clinical examination

Preoperative planning starts with the careful assessment of patient history, including a complete study of all available medical records mentioning any previous surgical treatments. The following aspects should be addressed in detail: actual pain, limitations in daily life, sports and recreational activities, and all previous and current treatments. All patients should be asked if they had any trauma, surgeries, concomitant diseases, or infections in the past. In patients with ankle stiffness and/or equinus contracture, it should be clarified whether the stiffness and/or contracture has progressed over the last few months. Patients with any of the aforementioned contraindications should be excluded.

The routine physical examination includes careful inspection of both lower extremities and observation of the patient while walking and standing.[28,29] The patient's neurovascular status should be evaluated; in particular, the integrity of the tibial nerve function should be proved. Alignment, deformities, and foot/ankle/hindfoot position are visually assessed (**Fig. 1**). In cases with a cavovarus deformity, the first ray is assessed to evaluate if a fixed plantar flexion is causing the hindfoot varus.[30] Muscular functional status and atrophy should be assessed, and special attention should be paid to possible tightness of the heel cord and function of plantar flexors, including posterior tibial muscle and flexor hallucis longus muscle.[31] Next, pain or tenderness on palpation is evaluated. Hindfoot and ankle stability is assessed manually with the patient sitting.[29,32] Finally, tibiotalar range of motion is measured in the sagittal plane (plantar flexion/dorsiflexion) and in the coronal plane (eversion/inversion). Ankle range

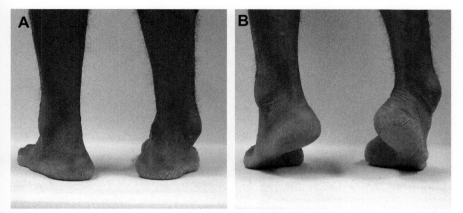

Fig. 1. Clinical assessment of the posterior view, showing a substantial varus deformity. (*A*) Standing position. (*B*) When moving into tip-toe position, the varus increases due to the fixed forefoot pronation (fixed first ray).

of motion is determined with a goniometer, which is placed along the lateral border of the leg and foot. All goniometer measurements are performed in the weight-bearing position as described by Lindsjö and colleagues.[33] To ensure the range of motion measurement is solely from the tibiotalar joint and not also in combination with the midfoot/hindfoot joints, it is recommended to use weight-bearing lateral radiographs in the position of maximal dorsiflexion and plantar flexion.[3,11,34,35]

Radiographic evaluation

As non–weight-bearing radiographs do not show the true extent of the deformity (**Fig. 2**), the routine radiographic evaluation should include bilateral weight-bearing anteroposterior and lateral views of the foot and ankle (**Fig. 3**A–C). For appropriate assessment of inframalleolar alignment, a hindfoot alignment view (Saltzman view) should be performed (**Fig. 3**D).[36,37] Weight-bearing radiographs should be used to identify and quantify degenerative changes, malposition, and deformities of the tibiotalar joint.[38] Furthermore, possible concomitant degenerative changes and/or deformities in the adjacent joints of the hindfoot and midfoot should be identified and assessed. Recently, the routine use of weight-bearing computed tomography was started to assess hindfoot alignment and the complexity of the degenerative changes of the hindfoot (**Fig. 4**).[39–41] Magnetic resonance imaging (MRI) is not routinely recommended. However, in some cases, this imaging may be helpful to evaluate possible tendon and muscular pathologies.[42]

Surgical Strategies

At the time of TAR, periarticular osteotomies are indicated when the preexisting deformities cannot sufficiently be addressed by correcting resection cuts, soft tissue releases (including ligaments, capsular, tendons), ligament reconstructions, and/or tendon transfers, for example, a stable and well-balanced ankle joint complex would not be achieved with all these measures.

Periarticular osteotomies

Periarticular correcting osteotomies have been shown to be the most successful treatment to balance a malaligned ankle with early stage OA while still preserving the ankle

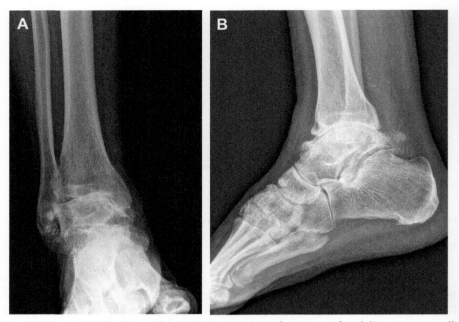

Fig. 2. Non–weight-bearing radiographs do not show the extent of malalignment, overall deformity, and joint destruction. (*A*) Anteroposterior (AP) view. (*B*) Lateral view.

joint.[19,20,43,44] However, despite the procedure's success, only a few studies report on its use in the treatment of advanced stage ankle OA where the malaligned ankle joint cannot be preserved and thus TAR is considered.[16,22,45–52] Periarticular osteotomies are divided into supramalleolar, intraarticular, and inframalleolar osteotomies.

A supramalleolar osteotomy is considered in cases where the origin of deformity is located above the ankle joint (**Fig. 5**). As a principle, it is done before replacement of the ankle. The procedure aims to translate the ankle joint to be in line with the weight-bearing axis and to normalize the direction of the force vector of the triceps surae, thereby realigning the hindfoot.[19,20,53] An open or closing wedge osteotomy on the medial or lateral side, or, in severe deformities, an anterior, domelike osteotomy can be considered to achieve a neutral TAS angle and/or to correct a pathologic slope of distal tibia (**Fig. 6**). The height of osteotomy is selected according to the CORA with the aim to move the longitudinal axis of the tibia to cross the tibiotalar joint at its center.

Performed as a stand-alone procedure or in addition to a tibial correcting osteotomy, a fibular osteotomy (**Fig. 7**) is considered when addressing a malpositioning that may hinder reduction of the talus, for example, shortening, lengthening, derotation, or abduction.[54] Used implants for internal fixation of osteotomies should not hinder the insertion of the components of the ankle (**Fig. 8**).

An osteotomy of the medial malleolus serves to release the medial ankle with severe varus deformities, where the tension of the deltoid ligament hinders the talus from being properly positioned within the ankle mortise, for example, when there is a persisting talar tilt at the end of an ankle replacement.[15,47]

In contrast to a supramalleolar correction, an inframalleolar osteotomy is considered after TAR if there is a persisting malalignment of the hindfoot (**Fig. 9**).

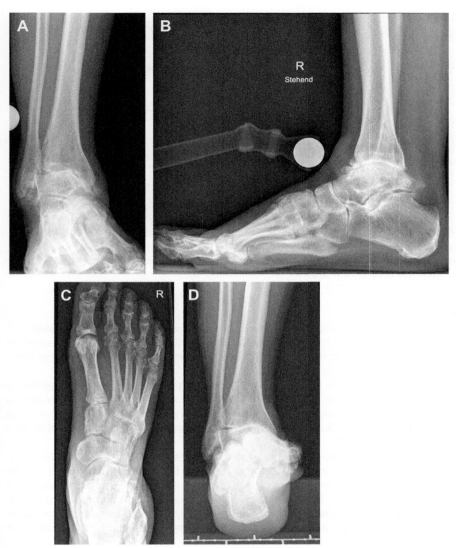

Fig. 3. Weight-bearing radiographs of same patient as **Fig. 2.** (*A*) AP view of the ankle, (*B*) lateral view of the foot and ankle, and (*C*) AP view of the foot. (*D*) Hindfoot alignment view (Saltzman view). These standard radiographs are taken bilaterally to assess the amount of deviation from the unaffected, contralateral foot and ankle and the overall deformity.

A calcaneal osteotomy aims to realign the hindfoot and normalize the direction of the force vector of the triceps surae. A lateral sliding osteotomy of the calcaneus (with or without lateral closing wedge)[55,56] or a Z-shaped calcaneal osteotomy[57,58] can be considered to achieve a neutral alignment of the hindfoot.

Osteotomies of the medial arch aim to realign the forefoot with the hindfoot. In the case of forefoot pronation, for example, a plantarflexed first metatarsal, a dorsal closing wedge osteotomy of first cuneiform is considered.[31,59]

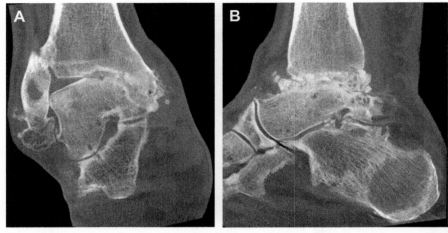

Fig. 4. Weight-bearing computed tomography scans are used to assess hindfoot alignment and the complexity of the degenerative changes of the hindfoot (same patient as **Fig. 2**). (*A*) AP view. (*B*) Lateral view shows a well-centralized talus beneath the tibia and significant degenerative changes at ankle joint.

Additional procedures

Although periarticular osteotomies are effective at balancing a malaligned ankles,[20,46] in some instances they may not be sufficient to achieve a stable and well-balanced ankle.[3,16,17,22,60] Therefore, additional procedures are often necessary for the long-term success of the replaced ankle.

A subtalar arthrodesis is considered to correct a fixed deformity,[61,62] stabilize a highly unstable joint, or address pain originating from progressive degenerative changes. In most instances, an interposition technique with the use of a bone graft should be considered to tighten the collapsed ligaments of the ankle joint complex.

A ligament reconstruction is considered to stabilize the talus in the corrected position within the ankle mortise.[32] Anatomic repair of the remaining ligaments can be augmented with the use of free tendon autografts, for example, plantaris tendon or semitendinosus tendon. If available, the use of allografts can also be considered. Although effective for stabilization of the ankle joint complex, tenodesis techniques should not be used, because they change the biomechanics and limit the motion of the ankle joint.

Tendon transfers are considered to restore and balance muscular forces. In cases with a dysfunctional peroneal brevis, a peroneus longus to peroneus brevis tendon transfer should be considered.[63]

Surgical Technique

The surgery can be performed under general or regional anesthesia. The patient is placed in a supine position, with the ipsilateral back of the patient lifted until a strictly upward position of the foot is obtained. A pneumatic tourniquet is applied on the ipsilateral thigh.

Fluoroscopic assessment should be done under anesthesia before surgery (**Fig. 10**). With passive manipulation and application of varus or valgus stress, the extent of correction of the talar position and the amount of lateral ankle instability can be assessed.

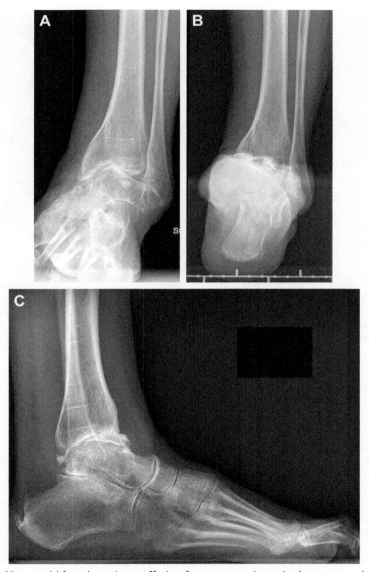

Fig. 5. A 68-year-old female patient suffering from progressive pain due to secondary OA in a severe varus deformity after a malunited ankle fracture at the age of 14 years. (*A*) The AP view shows a varus angulation of the distal tibia (TAS-angle) of 12° and a significantly shortened medial malleolus; the talus is tilted into varus by >20°. (*B*) The hindfoot alignment view confirms the varus malalignment of the hindfoot. (*C*) The lateral view shows the well-centralized position of the talus beneath the tibia.

If the varus deformity has its origin above the ankle joint, for example, in cases with a malunited tibial fracture or a tibia vara, a supramalleolar osteotomy is done first (see **Figs. 5–7**). Usually the osteotomy can be done through the same anterior approach, which later can be used for TAR. Although an opening wedge osteotomy

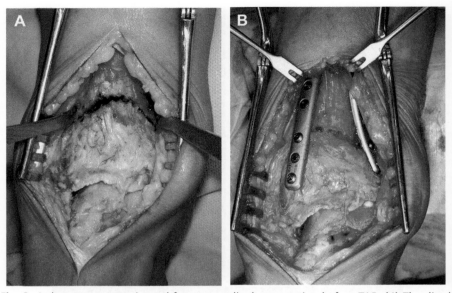

Fig. 6. A dome osteotomy is used for supramalleolar correction before TAR. (*A*) The distal tibia and the ankle joint are exposed through an anterior approach, and multiple drill holes are made along the circle. The distal tibia is then rotated into the desired neutral position. (*B*) Two plates are used for fixation.

is considered for minor corrections, a dome osteotomy is considered for a correction of more than 8°, because graft incorporation and bone healing would take too long for such an extended correction. In cases with a concomitant recurvatum deformity, the osteotomy is opened at its anterior aspect as well to realign the distal tibia in the sagittal plane. When fixating a plate, fixation should be done to avoid interfering with the subsequent TAR. After the supramalleolar correction, the anatomic axis of the tibia should cross the tibiotalar joint in its center in both the coronal and sagittal plane.

If TAR is still necessary after supramalleolar correction, the surgeons use the standard technique: the jig references the tuberosity of tibia for alignment in the coronal plane and the anterior tibial border for alignment in the sagittal plane (**Fig. 11**). If the talus cannot be reduced after insertion of all components, the medial ankle complex may be too tight or the fibula may be too long. Although an extended deltoid ligament release has been advocated by others,[16,22,52,60,64,65] the investigators prefer a flip osteotomy of the medial malleolus (**Fig. 12**).[15] The advantage of this technique is that the offset position of the medial malleolus is corrected toward normal; subsequently, the medial malleolus may guide the talus to its corrected position. Besides normalizing the external contours of the medial ankle, which may be beneficial when selecting shoe wear, the technique normalizes the pull of the deltoid ligament. This is not the case for Doets' lengthening osteotomy of the medial malleolus.[47] In addition, this vertical translational osteotomy weakens the medial shoulder of the ankle with the risk of a subsequent stress fracture.

Thereafter, lateral stability is tested with passive manipulation and varus stress. If the talus tilts into varus while applying varus stress, a ligament reconstruction is

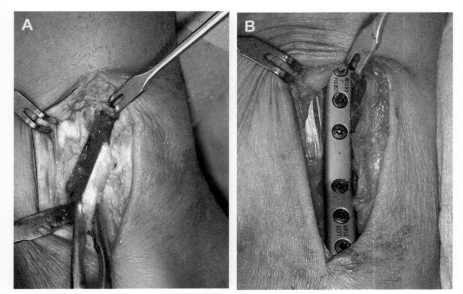

Fig. 7. The distal tibia cannot be moved without an osteotomy of the fibula. (*A*) The fibula is osteotomized with an oblique double cut, and the intermediate bone piece is removed. (*B*) Thereafter, the fibula is also fixed by a plate. Close attention is paid to the angulation at the osteotomy level.

completed with reattachment of torn ligaments to the fibula. This can be done through the anterior approach (**Fig. 13**) or by a separate lateral approach (**Fig. 14**).

As a next step, the heel position is carefully checked through comparison to the lower leg axis. If persistent varus deformity of the heel exists and can easily be corrected manually by applying eversion torque, a peroneus longus to peroneus brevis

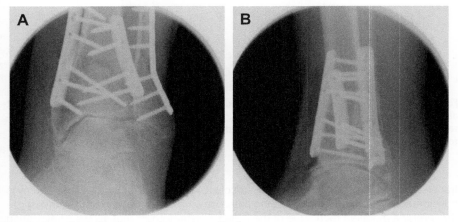

Fig. 8. The plate fixation of the supramalleolar correction must account for the space needed for the ankle prosthesis. (*A*) AP view; (*B*) lateral view.

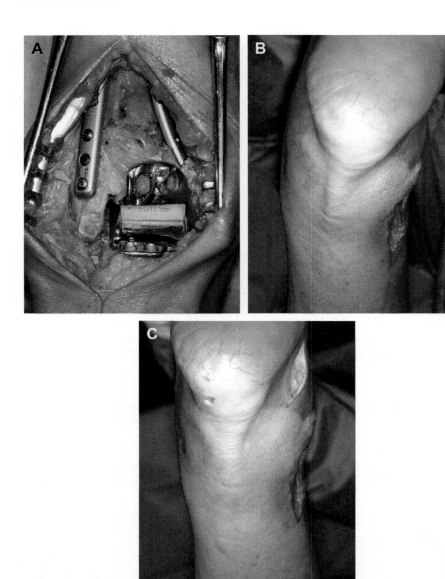

Fig. 9. (*A*) After the ankle prosthesis is inserted using the standard technique, the hindfoot alignment is checked clinically. (*B*) In this case, a valgus deformity has resulted from important supramalleolar correction. (*C*) After a medial sliding osteotomy of calcaneus, the hindfoot alignment has normalized.

transfer is done.[63] If the heel cannot be sufficiently corrected, a calcaneal osteotomy is considered.[66] Although a lateral sliding osteotomy has some limitations, the investigators prefer a modified technique of the Italian Z-osteotomy[58] that allows a valgization tilt and a lateral translation of the tuber calcanei.[57]

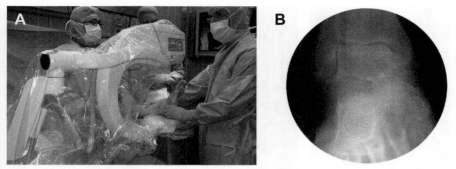

Fig. 10. Before starting the surgery, manual testing is used to determine whether the deformity is correctable. (*A*) Setup. (*B*) In this case, the talus can be reduced to neutral, indicating that the surgeon is dealing with a correctable deformity (same patient as **Fig. 2**).

Finally, forefoot alignment is checked by holding the foot in a neutral position. In the case of a plantar-flexed first ray, the first cuneiform or base of the first metatarsal is exposed through a dorsal approach. A closing wedge osteotomy is done to achieve appropriate correction of the forefoot.

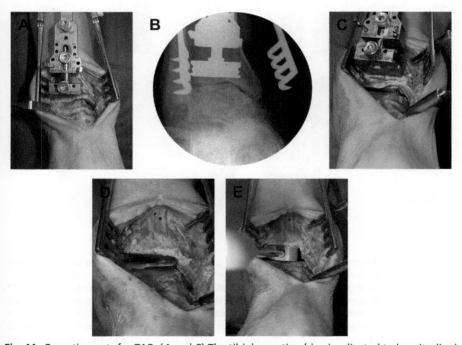

Fig. 11. Resection cuts for TAR. (*A* and *B*) The tibial resection bloc is adjusted to longitudinal axis of tibia which will typically result in a larger resection to lateral tibia. (*C*) Attention is paid to resect minimal bone on medial side. (*D*) Positioning of the foot in a strictly neutral position will ensure for a symmetrical cut on talar side. (*E*) After insertion of spacer, a subtle varus position is seen due to medial overstuff.

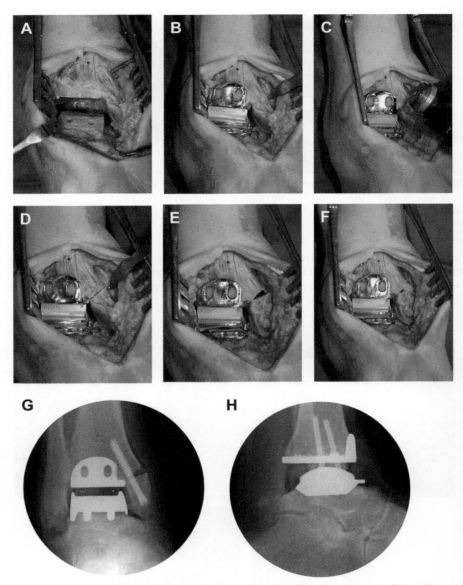

Fig. 12. Implant insertion and balancing of the ankle. (*A*) The resection cuts of the talus are finalized. (*B*) After insertion of the implants, the medial malleolus is in a medial deviation, leaving a substantial gap near the prosthesis and a distinct lateral opening of the ankle. (*C*) Therefore, an oblique osteotomy with a 45° to the longitudinal tibia axis is performed. (*D*) Osteotomy before mobilization of the medial malleolus. (*E*) The medial malleolus is turned to a neutral position and fixed by 2 percutaneous K-wires that serve to insert the cannulated screws. (*F*) Bone from resection of the tibia is used to fill the gap at the osteotomy site. (*G*) The AP-view under fluoroscopy shows the final situation with a well-balanced ankle. (*H*) Lateral view.

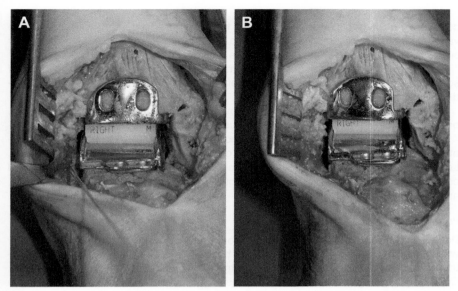

Fig. 13. Lateral ligament reconstruction through an anterior approach (same patient as **Fig. 2**). (*A*) A bony anchor is inserted into a hollow insertion site at the lateral ankle ligaments. (*B*) Final situation after reattachment of lateral ankle ligaments.

Complications

Intraoperative complications include neurovascular injuries. An important consideration, especially with acute corrections, is the posterior tibial nerve. Varus-to-valgus

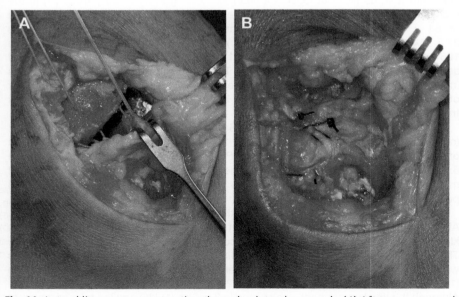

Fig. 14. Lateral ligament reconstruction through a lateral approach. (*A*) After exposure and debridement, the lateral ankle ligaments are taken by the sutures of a bony anchor. (*B*) Final situation after lateral ankle ligament reconstruction.

corrections stretch this nerve. Acute tarsal tunnel syndrome can originate from acute varus-to-valgus corrections. A prophylactic tarsal tunnel release may be indicated for such acute corrections, especially in cases with previous scarring.[67–70]

Perioperative wound-healing problems may result from inappropriate treatment of soft tissue during the surgery, the use of too bulky implants, and previous soft-tissue damage.

Over- or undercorrection may occur following inappropriate preoperative planning, or, if fluoroscopy is not used, for meticulous control of aimed cuts.

Delayed or nonunion of periarticular osteotomies may result from inappropriate fixation techniques or too aggressive loading of the leg in the early postoperative phase. Loss of correction may occur due to implant failure or inappropriately addressed concomitant problems, such as ligamentous incompetence, muscular dysfunction, and forefoot deformities.

Postoperative Management

Patients are placed in a below knee splint for 2 weeks followed by a removable walker with instructions to remain partially weight-bearing. In the case of additional interventions such as fusions or soft tissue reconstructions, a lower leg plaster may be used. Once bone healing is achieved (**Fig. 15**), usually after 8 weeks, full weight-bearing is permitted and a specific rehabilitation program is started. The program includes passive and active mobilization of the ankle, proprioception, coordination, gait improvement, and strength training.

RESULTS

In a consecutive cohort of 1244 primary TAR performed between 10/2000 and 12/2015, 140 ankles (18.4%) showed a preoperative varus hindfoot alignment associated with a varus tilt of at least $5°$ (mean $12° \pm 6°$ [range, $5°$-$35°$] varus tilt) in the mortise preoperatively. There were 98 male and 42 female patients with a mean age of 64 ± 10.7 years (range, 22–85 years). The mean body mass index was 27.5 ± 4.4 kg/m^2 (range, 17.8–40.5 kg/m^2). The cause of OA was posttraumatic in 106 ankles (75.7%), primary in 16 ankles (11.4%), systemic in 12 ankles (8.6%), and secondary/other reason in 6 ankles (4.3%). Two hundred fifty-two additional surgeries (mean 1.8 [range, 0–6] per ankle) were done at the time of TAR (**Table 1**). The number of additional surgeries was lower in the first 70 ankles treated than in the last 70 ankles treated.

The American Orthopedic Foot & Ankle Society hindfoot score increased from 37.2 (range, 7–70) preoperatively to 76.6 (range, 10–100) at the last follow-up, with a mean of 5.0 ± 3.4 years (range, 2.0–12.8 years). Pain on visual analog scale improved from 6.2 (range, 2–10) preoperatively to 1.8 (range, 0–8) postoperatively. The ankle range of motion improved from $29.6°$ (range, $2°$–$60°$) preoperatively to $32.7°$ (range, $10°$-$60°$) postoperatively.

A postoperative dislocation of the polyethylene insert occurred in 3 ankles (2.1%). After revision, all but one were stable, and further evolution was uneventful. In 16 ankles, a revision of a metallic component or conversion into arthrodesis was performed. The Kaplan-Meier Survival estimate was 78.5% at 10 years. A revision of components was done in 10 ankles (7.2%) due to either loosening (3 ankles, 2.1%), subsidence (1 ankle, 0.7%), malpositioning (3 ankles, 2.7%), or deep infection (3 ankles, 2.1%). Although the tibial component was revised in 2 ankles (1.4%) and the talar component in 1 ankle (0.7%), a revision of both components was performed in 7 ankles (5.0%). A conversion into an ankle arthrodesis was done in 6 ankles (4.3%).

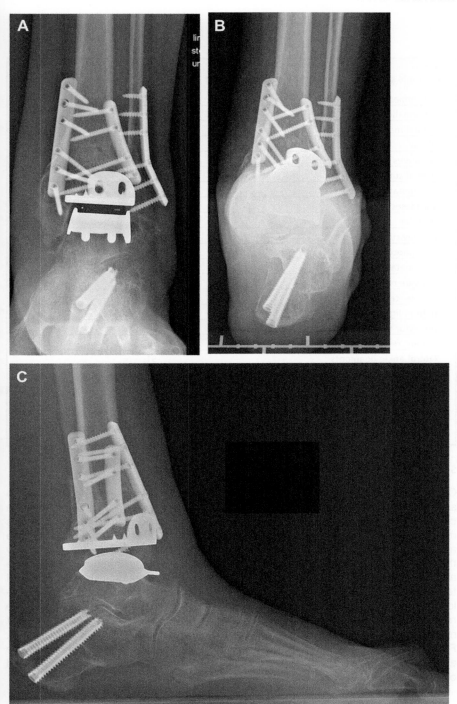

Fig. 15. Radiographic control after 8 weeks (same patient as **Fig. 5**). (*A*) The AP view shows a well-balanced ankle with advanced healing at the osteotomy site. (*B*) The alignment view reveals a well-aligned hindfoot after supra- and inframalleolar correction. (*C*) The lateral view shows a well-balanced ankle with stable implants.

Table 1 Additional surgeries during total ankle replacement		
Osteotomies		86
supramalleolar	10	
medial malleolus	36	
fibula	11	
calcaneus	8	
medial cuneiform	10	
first metatarsal	11	
Arthrodeses		38
subtalar	21	
talonavicular	10	
calcaneocuboid	3	
tarsometatarsal I	4	
Soft tissue releases		32
Achilles tendon lengthening	17	
deltoid ligament	11	
posterior tibial tendon	4	
Ligament reconstruction		53
lateral ankle ligaments	51	
medial ankle ligaments	2	
Tendon transfers		43
peroneus longus to peroneus brevis	34	
posterior tibial tendon	9	
Total		252

SUMMARY

Careful radiographic assessment of the talar position in all 3 planes is mandatory to successfully replace an end-stage osteoarthritic ankle joint associated with a concomitant major varus deformity. As correcting resection cuts for the prosthesis may not be able to restore proper position of the talus within the ankle mortise and provide overall stability of the ankle, additional osteotomies above or below the ankle or selective fusions may be necessary to obtain a well-balanced ankle and hindfoot joint complex. Besides lateral ligament reconstruction, peroneal tendon reconstruction or peroneus longus to peroneus brevis transfer and meticulous reorientation of the forefoot are mandatory for the long-term success of the replacement of a varus ankle. Overall, the key to success is to use all treatment modalities necessary to restore appropriate alignment of the hindfoot complex. From experience, the authors have learned to become more aggressive and use additional measures to balance the ankle. This strategy has led to an improved outcome.

ACKNOWLEDGMENTS

The authors thank Christine Schweizer (Clinic of Orthopedic Surgery, Kantonsspital Baselland, Liestal, Switzerland) for her help in preparing the manuscript and the figures. The authors also thank Maxwell Weinberg, BS (Department of Orthopedics, University of Utah, Salt Lake City, UT, USA) for his help with manuscript correction and editing review.

REFERENCES

1. Barg A, Bettin CC, Burstein AH, et al. Early clinical and radiographic outcomes of Trabecular Metal total ankle using transfibular approach. J Bone Joint Surg Am 2018;100(6):505–15.
2. Barg A, Wimmer MD, Wiewiorski M, et al. Total ankle replacement - indications, implant designs, and results. Dtsch Arztebl Int 2015;112(11):177–84.
3. Barg A, Zwicky L, Knupp M, et al. HINTEGRA total ankle replacement: survivorship analysis in 684 patients. J Bone Joint Surg Am 2013;95(13):1175–83.
4. Daniels TR, Mayich DJ, Penner MJ. Intermediate to long-term outcomes of total ankle replacement with the Scandinavian Total Ankle Replacement (STAR). J Bone Joint Surg Am 2015;97(11):895–903.
5. Daniels TR, Younger AS, Penner M, et al. Intermediate-term results of total ankle replacement and ankle arthrodesis: a COFAS multicenter study. J Bone Joint Surg Am 2014;96(2):135–42.
6. Hsu AR, Haddad SL. Early clinical and radiographic outcomes of intramedullary-fixation total ankle arthroplasty. J Bone Joint Surg Am 2015;97(3):194–200.
7. Lefrancois T, Younger A, Wing K, et al. A prospective study of four total ankle arthroplasty implants by non-designer investigators. J Bone Joint Surg Am 2017;99(4):342–8.
8. Nwachukwu BU, Mclawhorn AS, Simon MS, et al. Management of end-stage ankle arthritis: cost-utility analysis using direct and indirect costs. J Bone Joint Surg Am 2015;97(14):1159–72.
9. Queen RM, Sparling TL, Butler RJ, et al. Patient-reported outcomes, function, and gait mechanics after fixed and mobile-bearing total ankle replacement. J Bone Joint Surg Am 2014;96(12):987–93.
10. Ramaskandhan JR, Kakwani R, Kometa S, et al. Two-year outcomes of MOBILITY total ankle replacement. J Bone Joint Surg Am 2014;96(7):e53.
11. Rippstein PF, Huber M, Coetzee JC, et al. Total ankle replacement with use of a new three-component implant. J Bone Joint Surg Am 2011;93(15):1426–35.
12. Yi Y, Cho JH, Kim JB, et al. Change in talar translation in the coronal plane after mobile-bearing total ankle replacement and its association with lower-limb and hindfoot alignment. J Bone Joint Surg Am 2017;99(4):e13.
13. Arangio G, Rogman A, Reed JF 3rd. Hindfoot alignment valgus moment arm increases in adult flatfoot with Achilles tendon contracture. Foot Ankle Int 2009;30(11):1078–82.
14. Joo SD, Lee KB. Comparison of the outcome of total ankle arthroplasty for osteoarthritis with moderate and severe varus malalignment and that with neutral alignment. Bone Joint J 2017;99-B(10):1335–42.
15. Knupp M, Bolliger L, Barg A, et al. Total ankle replacement for varus deformity. Orthopade 2011;40(11):964–70 [in German].
16. Sung KS, Ahn J, Lee KH, et al. Short-term results of total ankle arthroplasty for end-stage ankle arthritis with severe varus deformity. Foot Ankle Int 2014;35(3):225–31.
17. Trajkovski T, Pinsker E, Cadden A, et al. Outcomes of ankle arthroplasty with preoperative coronal-plane varus deformity of 10 degrees or greater. J Bone Joint Surg Am 2013;95(15):1382–8.

18. Hintermann B, Knupp M, Barg A. Osteotomies of the distal tibia and hindfoot for ankle realignment. Orthopade 2008;37(3):212–8, 220–3. [in German].
19. Hintermann B, Knupp M, Barg A. Supramalleolar osteotomies for the treatment of ankle arthritis. J Am Acad Orthop Surg 2016;24(7):424–32.
20. Knupp M, Hintermann B. Treatment of asymmetric arthritis of the ankle joint with supramalleolar osteotomies. Foot Ankle Int 2012;33(3):250–2.
21. Hintermann B, Valderrabano V. Total ankle replacement. Foot Ankle Clin 2003; 8(2):375–405.
22. Jung HG, Jeon SH, Kim TH, et al. Total ankle arthroplasty with combined calcaneal and metatarsal osteotomies for treatment of ankle osteoarthritis with accompanying cavovarus deformities: early results. Foot Ankle Int 2013;34(1):140–7.
23. Barg A, Elsner A, Chuckpaiwong B, et al. Insert position in three-component total ankle replacement. Foot Ankle Int 2010;31(9):754–9.
24. Barg A, Knupp M, Henninger HB, et al. Total ankle replacement using HINTEGRA, an unconstrained, three-component system: surgical technique and pitfalls. Foot Ankle Clin 2012;17(4):607–35.
25. Hintermann B, Ruiz R, Barg A. Dealing with the stiff ankle: preoperative and late occurrence. Foot Ankle Clin 2017;22(2):425–53.
26. Alrashidi Y, Galhoum AE, Wiewiorski M, et al. How to diagnose and treat infection in total ankle arthroplasty. Foot Ankle Clin 2017;22(2):405–23.
27. Rosenbaum AJ, Dipreta JA. Classifications in brief: Eichenholtz classification of Charcot arthropathy. Clin Orthop Relat Res 2015;473(3):1168–71.
28. Apostle KL, Sangeorzan BJ. Anatomy of the varus foot and ankle. Foot Ankle Clin 2012;17(1):1–11.
29. Thevendran G, Younger AS. Examination of the varus ankle, foot, and tibia. Foot Ankle Clin 2012;17(1):13–20.
30. Coleman SS, Chesnut WJ. A simple test for hindfoot flexibility in the cavovarus foot. Clin Orthop Relat Res 1977;1(123):60–2.
31. Krause FG, Iselin LD. Hindfoot varus and neurologic disorders. Foot Ankle Clin 2012;17(1):39–56.
32. Klammer G, Benninger E, Espinosa N. The varus ankle and instability. Foot Ankle Clin 2012;17(1):57–82.
33. Lindsjö U, Danckwardt-Lilliestrom G, Sahlstedt B. Measurement of the motion range in the loaded ankle. Clin Orthop Relat Res 1985;199(1):68–71.
34. Hintermann B, Knupp M, Barg A. [Joint preserving surgery in patients with peritalar instability]. Fuss Sprungg 2013;11(4):196–206.
35. Hintermann B, Valderrabano V, Dereymaeker G, et al. The HINTEGRA ankle: rationale and short-term results of 122 consecutive ankles. Clin Orthop Relat Res 2004;424(1):57–68.
36. Barg A, Amendola RL, Henninger HB, et al. Influence of ankle position and radiographic projection angle on measurement of supramalleolar alignment on the anteroposterior and hindfoot alignment views. Foot Ankle Int 2015;36(11):1352–61.
37. Saltzman CL, El-Khoury GY. The hindfoot alignment view. Foot Ankle Int 1995; 16(9):572–6.
38. Linklater JM, Read JW, Hayter CL. Ch 3 Imaging of the foot and ankle. In: Saltzman CL, Anderson RB, editors. Mann's surgery of the foot and ankle. 9th edition. Philadelphia: Elsevier Saunders; 2014. p. 61–120.
39. Barg A, Bailey T, Richter M, et al. Weightbearing computed tomography of the foot and ankle: Emerging technology topical review. Foot Ankle Int 2017;39(3): 376–86.

40. Colin F, Horn Lang T, Zwicky L, et al. Subtalar joint configuration on weightbearing CT scan. Foot Ankle Int 2014;35(10):1057–62.
41. Krahenbuhl N, Tschuck M, Bolliger L, et al. Orientation of the subtalar joint: measurement and reliability using weightbearing CT scans. Foot Ankle Int 2016;37(1): 109–14.
42. Hintermann B. What the orthopaedic foot and ankle surgeon wants to know from MR Imaging. Semin Musculoskelet Radiol 2005;9(3):260–71.
43. Barg A, Saltzman CL. Single-stage supramalleolar osteotomy for coronal plane deformity. Curr Rev Musculoskelet Med 2014;7(4):277–91.
44. Pagenstert G, Knupp M, Valderrabano V, et al. Realignment surgery for valgus ankle osteoarthritis. Oper Orthop Traumatol 2009;21(1):77–87.
45. Brunner S, Knupp M, Hintermann B. Total ankle replacement for the valgus unstable osteoarthritic ankle. Tech Foot & Ankle 2010;9(4):165–74.
46. Deorio JK. Peritalar symposium: total ankle replacements with malaligned ankles: osteotomies performed simultaneously with TAA. Foot Ankle Int 2012;33(4): 344–6.
47. Doets HC, Van Der Plaat LW, Klein JP. Medial malleolar osteotomy for the correction of varus deformity during total ankle arthroplasty: results in 15 ankles. Foot Ankle Int 2008;29(2):171–7.
48. Gauvain TT, Hames MA, Mcgarvey WC. Malalignment correction of the lower limb before, during, and after total ankle arthroplasty. Foot Ankle Clin 2017;22(2): 311–39.
49. Hanselman AE, Powell BD, Santrock RD. Total ankle arthroplasty with severe preoperative varus deformity. Orthopedics 2015;38(4):e343–6.
50. Kim BS, Lee JW. Total ankle replacement for the varus unstable osteoarthritic ankle. Tech Foot & Ankle 2010;9(4):157–64.
51. Knupp M, Stufkens SA, Bolliger L, et al. Total ankle replacement and supramalleolar osteootomies for malaligned osteoarthritic ankles. Tech Foot & Ankle 2010;9(4):175–81.
52. Ryssman DB, Myerson MS. Total ankle arthroplasty: management of varus deformity at the ankle. Foot Ankle Int 2012;33(4):347–54.
53. Knupp M, Stufkens SA, Bolliger L, et al. Classification and treatment of supramalleolar deformities. Foot Ankle Int 2011;32(11):1023–31.
54. Hintermann B, Barg A, Knupp M. Corrective supramalleolar osteotomy for malunited pronation-external rotation fractures of the ankle. J Bone Joint Surg Br 2011;93(10):1367–72.
55. Barg A, Horterer H, Jacxsens M, et al. Dwyer osteotomy : Lateral sliding osteotomy of calcaneus. Oper Orthop Traumatol 2015;27(4):283–97 [in German].
56. Dwyer FC. Osteotomy of the calcaneum for pes cavus. J Bone Joint Surg Br 1959;41-B(1):80–6.
57. Knupp M, Horisberger M, Hintermann B. A new Z-shaped calcaneal osteotomy for 3-plane correction of severe varus deformity of the hindfoot. Tech Foot & Ankle 2008;7(2):90–5.
58. Malerba F, De Marchi F. Calcaneal osteotomies. Foot Ankle Clin 2005;10(3): 523–40.
59. Easley ME, Vineyard JC. Varus ankle and osteochondral lesions of the talus. Foot Ankle Clin 2012;17(1):21–38.
60. Queen RM, Adams SB Jr, Viens NA, et al. Differences in outcomes following total ankle replacement in patients with neutral alignment compared with tibiotalar joint malalignment. J Bone Joint Surg Am 2013;95(21):1927–34.

61. Kim BS, Knupp M, Zwicky L, et al. Total ankle replacement in association with hindfoot fusion: outcome and complications. J Bone Joint Surg Br 2010;92(11): 1540–7.
62. Usuelli FG, Maccario C, Manzi L, et al. Clinical outcome and fusion rate following simultaneous subtalar fusion and total ankle arthroplasty. Foot Ankle Int 2016; 37(7):696–702.
63. Kilger R, Knupp M, Hintermann B. Peroneus longus to peroneus brevis tendon transfer. Tech Foot & Ankle 2009;8(3):146–9.
64. Roukis TS. Tibialis posterior recession for balancing varus ankle contracture during total ankle replacement. J Foot Ankle Surg 2013;52(5):686–9.
65. Ryssman D, Myerson MS. Surgical strategies: the management of varus ankle deformity with joint replacement. Foot Ankle Int 2011;32(2):217–24.
66. Tennant JN, Carmont M, Phisitkul P. Calcaneus osteotomy. Curr Rev Musculoskelet Med 2014;7(4):271–6.
67. Bruce BG, Bariteau JT, Evangelista PE, et al. The effect of medial and lateral calcaneal osteotomies on the tarsal tunnel. Foot Ankle Int 2014;35(4):383–8.
68. Cody EA, Greditzer HGT, Macmahon A, et al. Effects on the tarsal tunnel following Malerba Z-type osteotomy compared to standard lateralizing calcaneal osteotomy. Foot Ankle Int 2016;37(9):1017–22.
69. Vanvalkenburg S, Hsu RY, Palmer DS, et al. Neurologic deficit associated with lateralizing calcaneal osteotomy for cavovarus foot correction. Foot Ankle Int 2016; 37(10):1106–12.
70. Walls RJ, Chan JY, Ellis SJ. A case of acute tarsal tunnel syndrome following lateralizing calcaneal osteotomy. Foot Ankle Surg 2015;21(1):e1–5.

Hindfoot Injuries
How to Avoid Posttraumatic Varus Deformity?

Stefan Rammelt, MD, PhD[a],*, Akaradech Pitakveerakul, MD[b]

KEYWORDS

• Talus • Calcaneus • Sustentaculum • Fracture • Malunion • Correction

KEY POINTS

• When treating talar neck and body fractures, adequate visualization of the talar neck via bilateral approaches is essential in avoiding rotatory or varus deformity.
• In cases of medial comminution of the talar neck, lag screws must be avoided and the use of single or double plates should be considered depending on fragment size.
• Impaction of the medial facet of the talus or calcaneus (sustentacular fractures) must be addressed to avoid hindfoot varus.
• A Schanz screw introduced into the calcaneal tuberosity is instrumental in realigning traumatic shortening and varus/valgus deformity of the heel.
• When using a lateral calcaneal plate, it must not be bent along its longitudinal axis.

INTRODUCTION

Posttraumatic varus deformities at the hindfoot lead to eccentric loading of the bones and joints with numerous potential subsequent problems, such as posttraumatic arthritis, stress fractures, peroneal tendon dislocation, ankle and subtalar instability or stiffness, and anterior ankle impingement.[1–4] Moreover, these conditions disturb the physiologic relationship of the ankle, hindfoot, and midfoot, thus leading to progressive foot and ankle deformities and overall functional limitation.[5,6] The optimal way to prevent these posttraumatic problems from happening is avoidance through awareness of possible pitfalls, and appropriate surgical planning and techniques. This article addresses surgical techniques to avoid varus malposition and

Disclosure: The authors do not have any relationship with a commercial company that has a direct financial interest in subject matter or materials discussed in this article or with a company making a competing product.
[a] University Center for Orthopaedics and Traumatology, University Hospital Carl-Gustav Carus at TU Dresden, Fetscherstrasse 74, Dresden 01307, Germany; [b] Department of Orthopaedic Surgery, Sirindhorn Hospital, Bangkok Metropolitan Administration, 20 Onnuch 90, Prawet, Bangkok 10250, Thailand
* Corresponding author.
E-mail address: strammelt@hotmail.com

Foot Ankle Clin N Am 24 (2019) 325–345
https://doi.org/10.1016/j.fcl.2019.02.006
1083-7515/19/© 2019 Elsevier Inc. All rights reserved.

foot.theclinics.com

reconstructive strategies for correction of posttraumatic varus after hindfoot injuries; that is, talar and calcaneal fractures.

TALAR FRACTURES
Mechanism of Injury

The talus has a unique anatomy and function. About two-thirds of its surface is covered by cartilage. Thus, significant forces are needed to break the strong subchondral bone of the talus.[7,8] Consequently, most fractures of the talar neck and body result from high-energy mechanisms such as a fall from a height or motor vehicle accidents; less than 10% result from indirect force.[9] A high percentage of these patients are polytraumatized or multiply injured.[9,10] The high variability of the talar fractures and their low incidence together with the high prevalence of accompanying injuries make the treatment of these injuries challenging.

The talar neck is a point of low resistance. Therefore, fractures of the talar neck account for about 45% of all talar fractures and are produced by decelerating forces with axial impaction.[9–11] According to biomechanical studies, the talus acts as a cantilever between the tibia and the calcaneus, and the sustentaculum tali acts as a lever arm while the foot is in dorsiflexion.[12] With the foot in plantarflexion, the more variable talar body fractures are thought to be produced by the same mechanism, whereas sagittal fractures of the talar dome seem to result from shearing forces.[12,13] Regularly, the impact of the sustentaculum tali at the time of injury leads to a comminution zone at the medial aspect of the talar neck and body.[14]

Most talar fractures are intra-articular and at a high risk of posttraumatic arthritis.[4–8,13–16] Fractures of the talar neck are extra-articular, but malunion invariably leads to posttraumatic rotational or varus deviation resulting in three-dimensional foot deformities with overload of the adjacent joints.[4,5] In particular, posttraumatic varus deformity is frequently encountered after talar neck and body fractures and can be avoided in most instances with adequate evaluation, reduction, and fixation.

Evaluation

Talar fractures are clinically evident with pain, swelling and ecchymosis over the ankle and hindfoot (**Fig. 1**). Range of motion at the ankle, subtalar, and midtarsal joints is restricted. However, the clinical diagnosis may be delayed in polytraumatized patients. For that reason, repeat physical examinations of unconscious patients in the intensive care unit are recommended.[10,17]

The clinical diagnosis is verified by standard anteroposterior and lateral views of the ankle. Furthermore, a computed tomography (CT) scan is mandatory in almost all talar fractures. CT imaging is essential for analyzing the exact fracture morphology and thus determining treatment, including surgical planning (**Fig. 2**). It may reveal occult central or peripheral (process) fractures and essential information like comminution zones.[7] In acute fracture-dislocations, CT scanning is deferred to after gross reduction of the main fragments.[18]

Nondisplaced fractures of the talar neck or body can be treated nonoperatively. The patients are mobilized on 2 crutches with sole contact for 8 to 10 weeks. Full weight bearing is allowed at the time of complete radiographic union, usually at 12 weeks. Radiographs are taken at 2 and 4 weeks to rule out secondary dislocation. Alternatively, stable internal fixation with minimal incision may allow early functional rehabilitation and reduce the risk of redislocation with malunion or nonunion.[7,19,20]

In order to avoid posttraumatic deformities, surgical treatment is recommended for all displaced talar fractures.[7] Nonoperative treatment of displaced talar neck and body

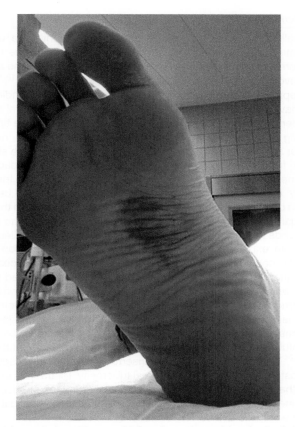

Fig. 1. Plantar ecchymosis in a 17-year-old female patient with talar body fracture.

fractures regularly leads to symptomatic malunion and nonunion.[1,5,21] Contraindications to open reduction include superficial soft tissue infections, advanced peripheral vascular disease, chronic venous insufficiency with skin ulceration, systemic immunodeficiency, and noncompliant patients. If open reduction is contraindicated in fracture-dislocations or severely displaced talar neck and body fractures, closed reduction under complete relaxation of the patient and percutaneous fixation may be attempted in order to avoid gross deformity.[18,22]

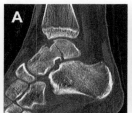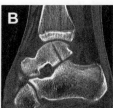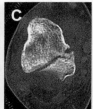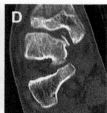

Fig. 2. (A) CT scans of the same patient as in **Fig. 1**. Typically, there is a comminution on the medial side and a (B) simple facture on the lateral side, as also seen on the (C) axial scan. (D) The coronal scan reveals impression of the medial talar dome.

Surgical Treatment Strategies

Inadequate visualization is a common cause for residual deformity after open reduction and internal fixation of talar fractures.[4,7] Bilateral approaches to the talar neck and body are therefore recommended to ensure anatomic reduction of the ankle and subtalar joints and avoid malalignment or malrotation at the talar neck.[14,18,19] Typically, an anteromedial approach starting over the medial malleolus and extending in a curved manner to the navicular tuberosity (**Fig. 3**A) is combined with a lateral approach. The latter is either performed as a slightly curved incision starting at the tip of the lateral malleolus running toward the sinus tarsi and lateral aspect of the talar neck (anterolateral approach) or alternatively as an oblique incision running along the skin crests over the sinus tarsi in front of the lateral malleolus (Ducroquet-Ollier approach). Soft tissue dissection is done from the floor of the sinus tarsi in order to preserve the blood supply to the talar body. On the medial side, the dissection must not extend beyond the sustentaculum tali in order not to injure the deltoid arterial branches within the deep portion of the deltoid ligament, which carries an important blood supply to the talar body.[19] If the fracture extends far into the talar body, an additional medial malleolar osteotomy provides adequate exposure. Infrequently, in cases of comminution of the lateral aspect of the talar dome, a lateral malleolar osteotomy becomes necessary.[22]

After identification, manipulation of the main fragments is alleviated with Kirschner wires (K-wires), which are used as joysticks to correct malrotation or malalignment of the displaced fragments.[14,18] This technique avoids the use of pointed reduction clamps, which need a larger exposure and potentially harm the cartilage.

An Arbeitsgemeinschaft für Osteosynthesefragen (AO) femoral or collinear foot distractor is a helpful tool to increase visualization of the tibiotalar, subtalar, and talonavicular joints.[23,24] The pins of distractor are inserted into the medial aspect of the tibial shaft and the posterior aspect of the calcaneal tuberosity. Distraction by a distractor is more effective than by manipulation with a K-wire or a Schanz pin because it can be steadily maintained, thus it allows comfortable manipulation. Application of the distractor on the medial side avoids varus stress.

The fragments of the talar dome and neck are anatomically reduced from posterior to anterior and from lateral to medial respectively (**Fig. 3**B). After reduction of the ankle and talonavicular joint via the medial approach, anatomic reduction and congruity of the subtalar joint are checked from lateral. Even if the talar neck appears anatomic on the medial side, malreduction in varus or tilting of the distal (head) fragment in supination or pronation with loss of contact of the main fragments on the lateral side has to be ruled out from the lateral approach (**Fig. 4**). Because the cortex is stronger on the lateral side and the sustentaculum impacts on the medial side of the talar neck, the

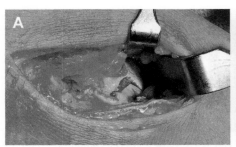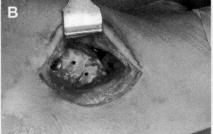

Fig. 3. (*A*) Anteromedial approach to the talar body. (*B*) Small fragments are fixed with resorbable pins (same patient as in **Figs. 1** and **2**).

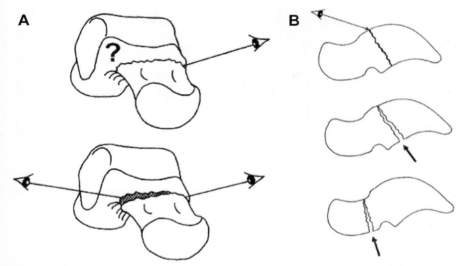

Fig. 4. (*A*) Bilateral approaches to the talar neck and body are essential to avoid varus malalignment or malrotation. (*B*) Reduction of the ankle joint is checked mostly via a medial approach, whereas the subtalar joint can only be evaluated via a lateral approach. *Arrows* represent directions of view. (*From* Cronier P, Talha A, Massin P. Central talar fractures–therapeutic considerations. Injury 2004;35(Suppl 2):SB16; with permission.)

lateral fracture is typically a simple one and control of reduction is therefore straightforward.

If a fracture gap or step-off is seen laterally, a varus deformity or malrotation of the talar neck in the horizontal plane needs to be corrected. Temporary fixation is achieved with a minimum of 2 K-wires introduced from the talar head close to the talonavicular joint surface into the talar body (**Fig. 5**). The quality of reduction is verified with intraoperative fluoroscopy in 3 projections (anteroposterior and lateral view of the ankle and a dorsoplantar view of the foot).

After anatomic reduction is ensured clinically and fluoroscopically, at least 2 small fragment screws (3.5–4.0 mm) are introduced perpendicular to the main fracture lines (**Fig. 6**). Depending on the size, location, and comminution of the fragments, fixation is

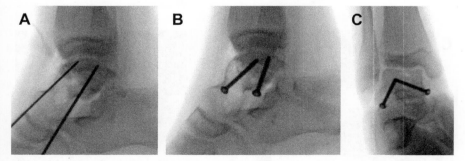

Fig. 5. (*A*) When anatomic reduction is confirmed fluoroscopically, (*B*) internal fixation is achieved with screws. (*C*) The lateral screw can be used as a lag screw because there is a simple fracture at the lateral talar body. The medial screw must not be lagged because this may induce varus malalignment because of the multiple fragmentation (same patient as in **Figs. 1–3**).

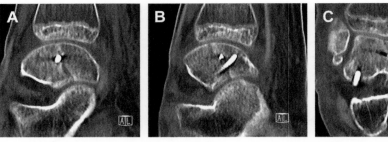

Fig. 6. (*A–C*) Postoperative CT scanning shows anatomic reduction of the joint surfaces and anatomic shape (same patient as in **Figs. 1–3** and **5**).

achieved with conventional, headless screws or small plates along the talar neck and body.[14,22,24,25]

When performing internal fixation, secondary displacement of the fracture should be avoided. First, in cases of medial comminution along the talar neck, any compression across the medial talar neck must be avoided otherwise shortening of the medial talar neck and varus malalignment in the horizontal plane resulting in forefoot adduction will result. Therefore, fully threaded positioning screws should be used medially. A compression screw may be used on the lateral side if there is a simple fracture (**Fig. 7**). Second, if the screw is inserted too tangentially at the talar head, the distal fragment may be pushed down by the screw head. The head therefore has to be countersunk in the talar head. The same is done if the screws have to be inserted near or through the joint surface.[19,22] To enhance stability, screws should be inserted in a convergent manner from medial and lateral.[22,23]

If there is extensive comminution of the medial part of the talar neck or if the talar head fragment is too small to contain a screw, an interlocking minifragment plate

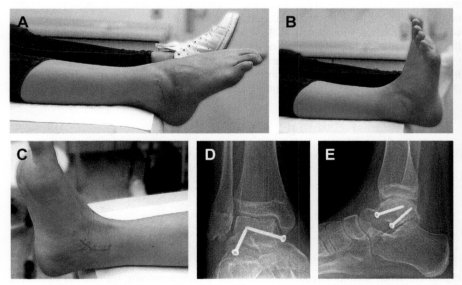

Fig. 7. (*A–C*) Uneventful scars and unrestricted function at 3 months postoperatively. (*D, E*) Radiographs at 3 months show consolidation of the fracture without signs of avascular necrosis or secondary displacement (same patient as in **Figs. 1–3, 5,** and **6**).

(2.0–2.7 mm) may be used for fixation of the medial wall (see **Figs. 9** and **10**). For multi-fragmentary fractures of the talar dome, and especially sagittal fractures through the body, headless screws are used for final fixation.[26,27] Small chondral or osteochondral fragments can be fixed with resorbable pins and fibrin glue or can be removed unless dependable to fixation.

Anatomic reduction and proper implant positioning are checked fluoroscopically in the standard anteroposterior and lateral projections. The talonavicular joint is assessed with a dorsoplantar view of the foot with a tube tilted 20° caudally. Subtalar joint congruity and lateral process alignment may additionally be checked with Brodén views.[28] Axial alignment of the talar neck can be assessed with the dorsoplantar and Canale views.[14,21]

Varus alignment of the hindfoot in the coronal plane may result from impaction of the medial facet of the subtalar joint through the sustentaculum tali of the calcaneus (**Fig. 8**). In these cases, the depressed medial facet has to be elevated (ie, brought down) and aligned to the anterior and medial facets of the calcaneus.[22] Local bone graft may be used to fill the defect and the fracture is buttressed with a plate from medial (**Figs. 9** and **10**).[14]

Management of Varus Malalignment

Varus malalignment is common after talar fractures.[4,5] Typical manifestations of malalignment at the talar neck are hindfoot varus, forefoot adduction, and shortening of the medial column.[4,5,29] Talar neck malalignment leads to eccentric loading of the peritalar joints, thus increasing the risk of posttraumatic arthritis.[30] After thorough clinical and radiographic assessment including bilateral weight-bearing radiographs of the foot and ankle, including a hindfoot alignment view, CT imaging, and MRI in case of suspected avascular necrosis (AVN), posttraumatic talar deformities can be classified as proposed previously (**Table 1**).

Varus malalignment can occur in any of the types of deformity. In type I to III deformities, anatomic reconstruction of the talus with joint preservation can be performed in

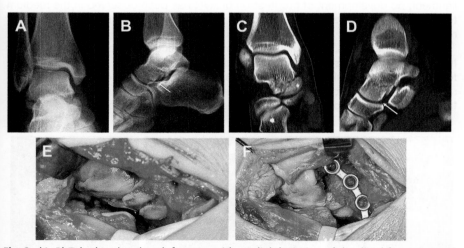

Fig. 8. (*A–D*) Talar head and neck fracture with medial deviation of the distal fragment and impression of the medial facet of the subtalar joint (*arrow* in *B, D*). Both result in varus malalignment if left unreduced. Intraoperative aspect of the medial impression (*E*) before and (*F*) after reduction toward the anteromedial facet of the calcaneus.

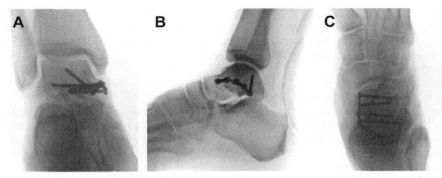

Fig. 9. (*A–C*) Fixation of the small talar head fragment and buttressing of the medial facet is achieved with a small medial plate (same patient as in **Fig. 8**).

reliable, active patients with adequate bone stock and intraoperative evidence of viable articular cartilage.[1,31,32] An extra-articular osteotomy at the talar neck is performed via the same approaches as for acute fracture treatment.[33] Correction of the varus deformity typically requires a medial opening wedge osteotomy with interposition of a bone graft.[1,29,32–34] If a nonunion is present (type II deformity), the former fracture is debrided from fibrous tissue, fracture callus, and subchondral sclerosis. After realignment of the talar neck, bone grafting is needed to enhance healing and avoid shortening of the medial column.[32,35]

In most cases, varus malalignment has resulted in manifest posttraumatic arthritis at the time of presentation. In these cases, corrective fusion of the ankle, subtalar, and/or talonavicular joint is the treatment of choice.[1,6] In the absence of AVN, total ankle replacement is an alternative treatment option.[4] In any case, fusion should be limited to the affected joints. Occasionally, the decision to reconstruct or fuse the joints is made at the time of surgery when directly assessing the cartilage status.[36] When reviewing the literature on joint-preserving talar osteotomies for posttraumatic malalignment, no development of progression of AVN has been observed in the medium term. However, posttraumatic arthritis has been noted in about half of the patients, necessitating fusion in about 15% of cases.[36,37]

In type IV malunions, correction of the deformity is accompanied with necrectomy, fusion of arthritic joints combined with autologous bone grafting of the resulting defects. In type V deformities, bone grafting and fusion can only be done after repeated radical debridements of all infected and necrotic bone, which may lead to subtotal talectomy. Whenever possible, the talonavicular joint should be preserved.[1,4]

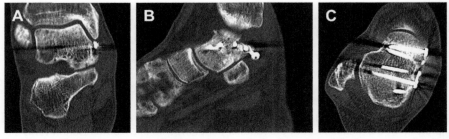

Fig. 10. (*A–C*) CT images at 4 months postoperatively show complete bony consolidation and anatomic reconstruction of the joint facets (same patient as in **Figs. 8** and **9**).

Table 1	
Classification of posttraumatic deformities after talar fractures	
Type I	Malunion/Joint Displacement
Type II	Nonunion with displacement
Type III	Types I/II with partial AVN
Type IV	Types I/II with complete AVN
Type V	Types I/II with septic AVN

Data from Rammelt S, Zwipp H. Corrective arthrodeses and osteotomies for post-traumatic hindfoot malalignment: indications, techniques, results. Int Orthop 2013;37(9):1707–17; and Zwipp H, Rammelt S. Posttraumatic deformity correction at the foot. Zentralbl Chir 2003;128:218–26, [in German].

CALCANEAL FRACTURES
Mechanism of Injury

Most calcaneal fractures originate from axial forces such as falls from a height or frontal crash motor vehicle accidents. More than three-fourths are the intra-articular type and the posterior facet of the calcaneus is involved in almost 90% of all intra-articular calcaneal fractures.[3,38,39] There are also increasing numbers of calcaneal fractures after low-velocity trauma, such as a misstep on a stair in elderly patients with osteoporosis.[40,41] The typical deformities include varus or valgus, broadening and shortening of the heel with loss of the longitudinal foot arch, tibiotalar, fibulocalcaneal, as well as soft tissue impingement.[1,3,42,43]

Evaluation

The clinical examination typically reveals pain, swelling, hematoma, and tenderness around the hindfoot. Visible deformities and axial deviations are noted. The patients are unable to bear weight on the heel. Blister formation and compartment syndrome of the foot may develop within a few hours.[44]

Standard radiographs include lateral, anteroposterior, and axial projections of the hindfoot (**Fig. 11**). If a displaced fracture is seen, lateral views of the unaffected

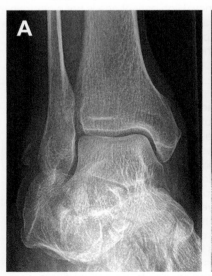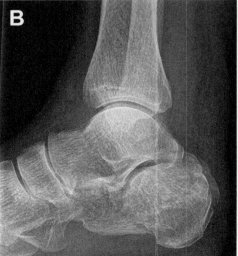

Fig. 11. (*A*) Anteroposterior and (*B*) lateral radiograph showing a displaced intraarticular fracture.

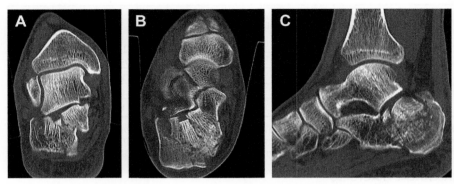

Fig. 12. (A) Axial, (B) sagittal, and (C) coronal CT scans revealing a Sanders type 3 fracture with multiple fragmentation of the subtalar joint and additional bulging of the lateral calcaneal wall (same patient as in **Fig. 11**).

calcaneus are useful to measure the individual normal values of Böhler and Gissane angles.[38] If an intra-articular fracture is suspected, CT scanning (**Fig. 12**) is essential to precisely analyze the fracture morphology for making the indication for surgery and preoperative planning.[3,38,45]

The ideal treatment of calcaneal fractures is still a matter of debate, which is beyond the scope of this review.[46] Many investigators agree that displaced intra-articular fractures should be reduced to avoid hindfoot deformities and posttraumatic subtalar arthritis.[1–3,38–53] Clinical and biomechanical studies suggest that surgical reduction should be pursued in patients with a joint step-off of greater than or equal to 2 mm, a gap of greater than 3 mm, and significant extra-articular fractures; that is, a hindfoot varus or valgus deformity greater than 10° and those with significant flattening, broadening, or shortening of the heel as well as bony prominences at the calcaneal tuberosity.[54–60]

Systemic contraindications for open reduction include severe neurovascular insufficiency, poorly controlled insulin-dependent diabetes mellitus, noncompliance, and severe systemic disorders with immunodeficiency. High patient age is not a contraindication to surgery because favorable results can be obtained in active patients more than 65 years old.[40,41,52] If surgical treatment is chosen, every effort should be made to anatomically reconstruct both the overall calcaneal geometry and the joint surfaces.[46]

Surgical Treatment Strategies

Choice of approaches
The best approach to a displaced calcaneal fracture is determined individually by the severity of injury, soft tissue conditions, time of patient presentation, comorbidities, and surgeon preference.[46] Pros and cons have to be weighed in every scenario.

The extended lateral approach (**Fig. 13**) allows good visualization of the lateral wall, the posterior facet, the sinus tarsi, and the anterior process including the calcaneocuboid joint.[38,42,45] It includes raising of a full-thickness fasciocutaneous flap from the lateral calcaneal wall, careful retraction of the peroneal tendons within their sheaths, and respecting the course of the sural nerve and the lateral calcaneal artery.[61] Because this approach is associated with a high risk of wound healing problems and postoperative scarring, less extensile approaches have been used. In particular, a small oblique approach directly over the sinus tarsi has become increasingly popular over the recent years.[60,62,63] The subtalar joint is accessed directly from the sinus tarsi but reduction of the overall shape of the calcaneus has to be judged fluoroscopically.[60] This approach can also be extended toward the calcaneocuboid joint.[58] Apart

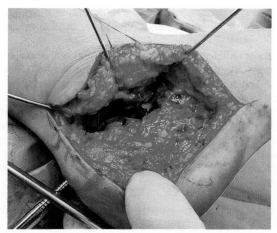

Fig. 13. Extensile lateral approach to the calcaneus. Note the Schanz screw in the tuberosity for manipulation of this fragment. K-wires are introduced to gently and continuously retract the soft tissue flap (same patient as in **Figs. 11** and **12**).

from temporary percutaneous fixation for patients with a critical overall condition or contraindication to extensile approaches,[10,58,64] a purely percutaneous fixation is most useful in selected patients with less severe fracture patterns.[65] This technique is particularly advised in cases of extra-articular and simple intra-articular fractures with the posterior facet being displaced as a whole, as in Sanders IIC fractures,[65,66] as well as an intra-articular fractures with just 1 displaced fracture line across the sub-talar joint (Sanders IIA and IIB). In the latter, arthroscopic control of reduction is advised.[67,68] With proper surgical technique, less invasive and percutaneous approaches significantly reduce the risk of soft tissue complications without compromising on the quality of reduction, whereas inadequate visualization or fixation may lead to improper reduction or secondary loss of reduction.[64,65,68]

In isolated fractures of the sustentaculum tali, a small medial approach directly over the palpable sustentaculum is performed.[69] The neurovascular bundle lies well plantar to the approach, whereas the posterior tibial, flexor digitorum longus, and flexor hallucis longus tendons are held away with vessel loops. If not reduced and fixed adequately, sustentacular fractures may lead to loss of height of the medial facet, resulting hindfoot varus and arthritis of the medial subtalar joint.[4,18,69]

Reduction techniques

For most types of calcaneal fractures, introduction of a Schanz screw into the tuberosity is helpful to realign the position of the calcaneal tuberosity, which defines the overall hindfoot alignment.[38,45] The patient is placed on the noninjured side on a radiolucent operating table. A 6.5-mm cancellous Schanz screw with handle is applied percutaneously to loosen the impacted articular fragments and thus allow better visualization of the displaced subtalar joint (see **Fig. 13**). Simultaneously, it can be used to correct any varus or valgus position by introduction from either the posterior or lateral aspect of the tuberosity.[38,39,42] This Westhues/Essex-Lopresti maneuver is also most helpful in minimally invasive and percutaneous reduction of displaced intra-articular calcaneal fractures.[62,65,66]

When using an extended lateral approach, the lateral calcaneal wall and a separate lateral joint fragment are held away. The subtalar joint is then reduced stepwise from medial to lateral starting with the sustentacular fragment.[38,70] In cases of comminuted fractures of the medial facet, an additional medial approach is used, as described earlier.[22,69]

To reconstruct the medial wall, the tuberosity fragment is pulled downward and medially beneath the sustentaculum. An elevator is applied as a lever between these two fragments.[58,70] The fragments are fixed to each other temporarily with K-wires.

To visually check the joint surface, any K-wires crossing the subtalar joint have to be removed and the heel brought into a slight varus position. If an intra-articular step-off is found, repeated joint reduction should be made. After ensuring exact reduction, a screw is inserted parallel to the joint into the sustentaculum to stabilize the articular portion of the calcaneus. Fluoroscopic Brodén views showing the various parts of the subtalar joint are useful for intraoperative assessment of joint reconstruction and screw placement.[28]

The tuberosity fragment is then reduced to the reconstructed subtalar joint block. Residual loss of heel height and varus or valgus deformity of the calcaneus is corrected at this stage by using the inserted Schanz screw as a lever. The fragments are temporarily fixed with K-wires (**Fig. 14**).

In case of remaining incongruities at the calcaneocuboid joint, the incision is extended distally from either the sinus tarsi or extended lateral approach to provide adequate visibility and allow congruent reduction of this joint.[58]

The lateral calcaneal wall is then folded back and should fit with the other fragments in case of anatomic reduction. Restoration of the anatomic shape of the calcaneus is checked fluoroscopically.

When using a sinus tarsi approach, the sequence of reduction of the main fragments is exactly the same.[46,58,62,67] The joint fragments can be seen and manipulated directly from above. With both extensile and less extensive approaches, visualization of all parts of the subtalar joint may be difficult. In these cases, open (dry) subtalar arthroscopy is most useful in detecting residual incongruities or intra-articular implants.[48,58]

Internal fixation

When using an extensile lateral approach, internal fixation is achieved with a single lateral plate that displays the anatomic features of the calcaneus, providing support

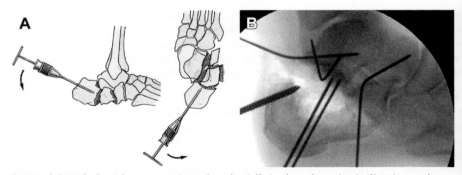

Fig. 14. (*A*) With the Schanz screw introduced axially in the tuberosity, inclination and varus or valgus deformity can be corrected (Westhues/Essex-Lopresti maneuver). (*B*) In a first step, the fragments are loosened and the tuberosity is reduced beneath the sustentacular fragment with the help of the Schanz screw and direct leverage. This step restores the medial wall and makes way for reduction of the lateral joint fragments. Temporary fixation is achieved with K-wires (same patient as in **Figs. 11–13**). ([A] *From* Rammelt S, Amlang M, Barthel S, et al. Minimally-invasive treatment of calcaneal fractures. Injury 2004;35(2 Suppl):58, Elsevier; with permission.)

to the tuberosity, the thalamic portion, the posterior joint facet, and the anterior process. Many investigators use interlocking, polyaxial plates to avoid secondary loss of correction, but there is no evidence that nonlocking plates are inferior.[38,42,45,49,52,70–73] Irrespective of its design, the plate should never be bent along the longitudinal axis in order to avoid varus deformity of the heel (**Fig. 15**). Because the lateral wall of the calcaneus is straight, any residual bowing of the lateral wall indicates malreduction and should be corrected rather than bending the plate. A prominent peroneal tubercle is removed or flattened to allow the plate to fit closely to the lateral calcaneal wall.

In general, a minimum of 2 screws should be directed into the sustentaculum tali, the tuberosity, and the anterior process.[38] One or 2 additional screws may be placed freely outside the plate in order to obtain ideal positioning into the sustentaculum tali, a severely displaced anterior process, or anterior facet fragment.[52] If a locking plate is used, 1 or 2 conventional screws should be placed first to bring the plate close to the bone, thus increasing stability by friction and avoiding soft tissue impingement from plate protrusion.[73] After plate fixation, all K-wires and the Schanz screw are removed (**Figs. 16** and **17**).

When using a sinus tarsi approach, definite fixation is achieved with percutaneous screws, an intramedullary nail with locking screws, or a small plate placed via the approach and tunneled beneath the peroneal tendons.[58,60,62,74,75]

Fractures of the Sustentaculum Tali

To avoid varus in sustentacular fractures, the original height of the sustentaculum has to be restored.[69] The sustentaculum tali, carrying the medial facet of the subtalar joint, is situated superior to the anterior part of the posterior facet of the calcaneus.[22] Therefore, if the contour of the strong cortical bone of the sustentaculum does not overlap with the posterior facet in a lateral radiographic view, the height of the sustentaculum is not adequate (**Fig. 18**).

As with fractures of the medial subtalar facet of the talus, if the height of the subtalar medial facet of the calcaneus is not restored, a varus malunion of the hindfoot is inevitable.[22] The sustentaculum is approached via a small, direct medial incision.[43] The

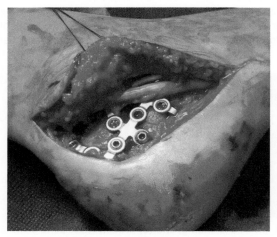

Fig. 15. Interlocking calcaneal plate in situ. The plate must not be bent along the lateral wall in order to avoid varus (same patient as in **Figs. 11–14**).

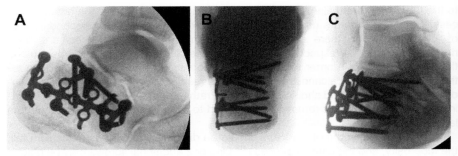

Fig. 16. (*A*) Lateral, (*B*) axial, and (*C*) Brodén view of the calcaneus after open reduction and plate fixation (same patient as in **Figs. 11–15**).

sustentacular fragment is identified and the fracture is cleared from debris. Intercalary fragments are fixed to the (lateral) calcaneal body or discarded if not amenable to internal fixation. The joint facet of the sustentaculum is then lifted up and aligned toward the corresponding medial facet of the talus (**Fig. 19**). After clinical and fluoroscopic control of reduction of the medial joint facet, the sustentacular fragment is fixed with 3.5-mm cortical screws along its axis.[58,69,76] According to the anatomy of the calcaneus, the screws are directed plantarly and posteriorly (**Fig. 20**).

Management of Varus Malalignment

Although operative treatment even in the best of hands does not guarantee a good outcome, nonoperative management or inadequate surgical reduction and fixation of displaced intra-articular calcaneal fractures regularly results in painful malunions or nonunions with the development of posttraumatic arthritis and severe functional deficits.[1–3,6,53,77–80]

Residual step-offs in the subtalar joint or severe cartilage damage at the time of injury regularly lead to posttraumatic subtalar arthritis. The typical posttraumatic deformities include loss of calcaneal height, heel broadening, hindfoot varus or valgus, lateral shift of the heel after fracture-dislocations, and even talar tilt within the ankle mortise.[1–3] These bony deformities lead to multiple soft tissue problems such as painful callosities or ulcerations at overloaded portions of the heel, impingement and/or subluxation of the peroneal tendons at the displaced lateral calcaneal wall, flexor hallucis longus entrapment along a displaced medial wall or sustentaculum tali,

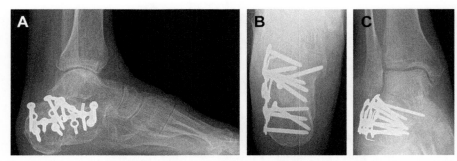

Fig. 17. (*A*) Lateral, (*B*) axial standing, and (*C*) Brodén views at 10 years showing anatomic alignment and joint congruity with minimal signs of posttraumatic arthritis (same patient as in **Figs. 11–16**).

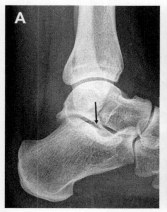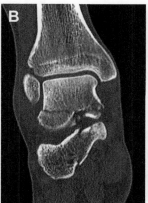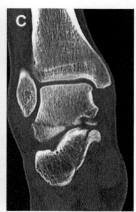

Fig. 18. (*A*) Lateral view of a sustentacular fracture combined with a talar body fracture. Note the irregular contour of the sustentaculum (*arrow*), which does not overlap with the contour of the lateral facet because of the impression. (*B*) Coronal CT scans show impression of both the sustentaculum tali and the medial facet of the talus. (*C*) Failure to reconstruct the original height on the medial side inevitably results in varus malalignment at the hindfoot.

fibulocalcaneal abutment with chronic peroneal dislocation or laceration in malunited fracture-dislocations, and sural or posterior tibial neuritis.[1–3,6,46,77–81]

Therefore, correction of the bony malunion is supplemented by various soft tissue balancing, include Achilles tendon lengthening, tenolysis of the peroneal tendons and superior peroneal retinaculum reconstruction, and tenolysis and/or lengthening of the flexor hallucis longus tendon.[1,22]

Symptomatic malunions require a precise preoperative assessment of the deformity before surgery. To provide a guideline for surgical correction, Zwipp and Rammelt[31] have proposed a simple classification including 5 types of typical posttraumatic calcaneal malunions. More recently,[1] a type 0 was added to describe any deformity without symptomatic subtalar arthritis including extra-articular deformities (**Table 2**). The latter is also compatible with the classification provided by Stephens and Sanders.[80] An isolated varus deformity would be classified as type II or type 0 if no signs of posttraumatic arthritis are present, mainly in extra-articular deformities. However, varus (or valgus) malalignment can be combined with any other deformity as in types III to V.

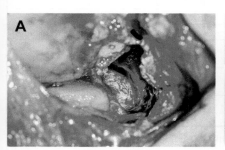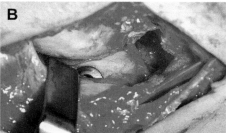

Fig. 19. (*A*) Intraoperative aspect of the sustentacular approach showing impression of the medial facet of both the talus and calcaneus resulting in gaping of the joint space. (*B*) After lifting up the sustentaculum and buttressing the medial facet of the talus, congruity of the medial aspect of the subtalar joint is restored (same patient as in **Fig. 18**).

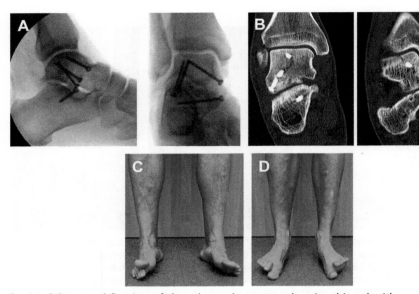

Fig. 20. (*A*) Internal fixation of the talus and sustentaculum is achieved with screws (*left panel*: lateral view, *right panel*: ap view). Note that the contour of the sustentaculum now overlaps with the lateral facet of the subtalar joint. (*B*) Postoperative CT scanning showing restoration of the height of both the sustentaculum and talus with congruent subtalar joint. (*C*, *D*) Free range of motion at the subtalar and midtarsal joints is seen 6 months postoperatively (same patient as in **Figs. 18** and **19**).

In type 0 malunions, an extra-articular or intra-articular joint-preserving corrective osteotomy may be performed in compliant patients with good bone quality.[82,83] With an isolated lateral exostosis, decompression of the lateral wall and exostectomy has been reported with good results.[80,81] Extra-articular varus deformity is treated with a lateralizing and closing wedge osteotomy of the calcaneal tuberosity below the peroneal tendons.[1]

Table 2 Classification of calcaneal malunions		
Type	**Characteristics**	**Treatment Options**
0	Any deformity without subtalar arthritis	Joint-preserving osteotomy
I	Subtalar arthritis without deformity	In situ subtalar fusion
II	Additional hindfoot varus/valgus	Subtalar bone block fusion (+osteotomy)
III	Additional loss of height	Subtalar distraction bone block fusion (+osteotomy)
IV	Additional lateral translation of the tuberosity	Corrective osteotomy along the former fracture and subtalar fusion
V	Additional talar tilt at the ankle joint	Ankle revision, corrective osteotomy/ subtalar fusion

The quality of the deformity can be encoded with an additional letter: A, solid malunion; B, nonunion; C, necrosis.

Data from Rammelt S, Zwipp H. Corrective arthrodeses and osteotomies for post-traumatic hindfoot malalignment: indications, techniques, results. Int Orthop 2013;37(9):1707–17; and Zwipp H, Rammelt S. Posttraumatic deformity correction at the foot. Zentralbl Chir 2003;128:218–26, [in German].

However, subtalar arthritis has developed in most calcaneal malunions at the time of presentation. Type I malunions with painful subtalar arthritis are treated successfully with subtalar in situ fusion, accompanied by lateral wall decompression in case of painful exostosis. Both procedures may be performed arthroscopically if no implant removal is needed.[84,85]

Type II malunions are treated with corrective subtalar fusion. Varus or valgus malalignment is corrected by either asymmetric joint resection or application of wedge-shaped bone blocks in mild deformities.[22] With considerable varus deformity (approximately >15°), tension of the deltoid ligament and the medial soft tissue typically prevents correction through the subtalar joint. In these cases, a lateral closing wedge osteotomy of the calcaneus is added to the subtalar fusion.[1,80]

Type III malunions are corrected with a subtalar distraction arthrodesis with bone block to reestablish heel height and relieve the subsequent anterior tibiotalar impingement.[1,2,6,77] An additional corrective osteotomy may be required for severe malalignment of the tuberosity. Type IV malunions represent malunited fracture-dislocations of the calcaneus with the tuberosity fragment displaced beneath the distal fibula. These deformities can be corrected by an osteotomy along the former fracture plane and additional subtalar fusion with bone grafting in case of remaining defects.[1,79] In type V malunions, talar tilt in the ankle requires an additional anterior approach with careful debridement of all intervening tissue and revision of the ankle mortise followed by realignment of the talus and calcaneus and corrective subtalar fusion via bilateral approaches.[1,22] Necrosis and infection require repeat debridements and secondary bone and soft tissue reconstruction.[86]

SUMMARY

Hindfoot injuries may be life-changing events for affected patients. They require a thorough assessment and individualized treatment approach after precise preoperative planning. Failure to reconstruct hindfoot anatomy results in complex three-dimensional foot deformities. Posttraumatic varus deformity can result from failure to restore the length of the medial aspect of the talus after talar neck and body fractures with medial comminution. The use of compression screws should be avoided in these cases. In the presence of calcaneal fractures it is essential to correct any malposition of the calcaneal tuberosity, which defines the overall shape of the calcaneus. The lateral wall must be straight after internal fixation. If a lateral plate is used, it should not be bent along its axis. In both talar and calcaneal fractures, impression of the medial aspect leads to varus malalignment of the hindfoot if not restored; this applies to fractures of the medial subtalar facet of the talus and the sustentaculum tali. Symptomatic malunions are treated with corrective osteotomies or corrective fusions depending on the degree of arthritis at the time of presentation.

REFERENCES

1. Rammelt S, Zwipp H. Corrective arthrodeses and osteotomies for post-traumatic hindfoot malalignment: indications, techniques, results. Int Orthop 2013;37(9): 1707–17.
2. Sangeorzan BJ, Hansen ST Jr. Early and late posttraumatic foot reconstruction. Clin Orthop Relat Res 1989;243:86–91.
3. Sanders R, Rammelt S. Fractures of the calcaneus. In: Coughlin MJ, Saltzman CR, Anderson JB, editors. Mann's surgery of the foot & ankle. 9th edition. St. Louis: Elsevier; 2013. p. 2041–100.

4. Rammelt S, Winkler J, Grass R, et al. Reconstruction after talar fractures. Foot Ankle Clin 2006;11(1):61–84, viii.
5. Daniels TR, Smith JW, Ross TI. Varus malalignment of the talar neck. Its effect on the position of the foot and on subtalar motion. J Bone Joint Surg Am 1996; 78(10):1559–67.
6. Rammelt S, Grass R, Zawadski T, et al. Foot function after subtalar distraction bone-block arthrodesis. A prospective study. J Bone Joint Surg Br 2004;86(5): 659–68.
7. Rammelt S, Zwipp H. Talar neck and body fractures. Injury 2009;40(2):120–35.
8. Lindvall E, Haidukewych G, DiPasquale T, et al. Open reduction and stable fixation of isolated, displaced talar neck and body fractures. J Bone Joint Surg Am 2004;86-A:2229–34.
9. Zwipp H. Severe foot trauma in combination with talar injuries. In: Tscherne H, Schatzker J, editors. Major fractures of the pilon the talus and the calcaneus. New York: Springer-Verlag; 1993. p. 123–35.
10. Rammelt S, Biewener A, Grass R, et al. Foot injuries in the polytraumatized patient. Unfallchirurg 2005;108:858–65.
11. Peterson L, Goldie IF, Irstam L. Fracture of the neck of the talus. A clinical study. Acta Orthop Scand 1977;48:696–706.
12. Peterson L, Romanus B, Dahlberg E. Fracture of the collum tali-an experimental study. J Biomech 1976;9:277–9.
13. Sneppen O, Christensen SB, Krogsoe O, et al. Fracture of the body of the talus. Acta Orthop Scand 1977;48:317–24.
14. Rammelt S, Winkler J, Zwipp H. Osteosynthesis of central talar fractures. Oper Orthop Traumatol 2013;25:525–41.
15. Vallier HA, Nork SE, Barei DP, et al. Talar neck fractures: results and outcomes. J Bone Joint Surg Am 2004;86-A:1616–24.
16. Vallier HA, Nork SE, Benirschke SK, et al. Surgical treatment of talar body fractures. J Bone Joint Surg Am 2003;85-A:1716–24.
17. Metak G, Scherer MA, Dannöhl C. Missed injuries of the musculoskeletal system in multiple trauma-a retrospective study. Zentralbl Chir 1994;119:88–94.
18. Rammelt S, Bartoníček J, Park KH. Traumatic injury to the subtalar joint. Foot Ankle Clin 2018;23:353–74.
19. Cronier P, Talha A, Massin P. Central talar fractures–therapeutic considerations. Injury 2004;35(Suppl 2):SB10–22.
20. Schulze W, Richter J, Russe O, et al. Surgical treatment of talus fractures: a retrospective study of 80 cases followed for 1-15 years. Acta Orthop Scand 2002; 73(3):344–51.
21. Canale ST, Kelly FB Jr. Fractures of the neck of the talus. J Bone Joint Surg Am 1978;60:143–56.
22. Zwipp H, Rammelt S. Tscherne Unfallchirurgie: Fuss. New York: Springer; 2014.
23. Fortin PT, Balazsy JE. Talus fractures: evaluation and treatment. J Am Acad Orthop Surg 2001;9(2):114–27.
24. Rammelt S, Schepers T. Chopart injuries: when to fix and when to fuse? Foot Ankle Clin 2017;22:163–80.
25. Fleuriau Chateau PB, Brokaw DS, Jelen BA, et al. Plate fixation of talar neck fractures: preliminary review of a new technique in twenty-three patients. J Orthop Trauma 2002;16:213–9.
26. Wheeler DL, McLoughlin SW. Biomechanical assessment of compression screws. Clin Orthop Relat Res 1998;(350):237–45.

27. Bretschneider H, Rammelt S. Combined ipsilateral fracture of the pilon tibiale, talar body and calcaneus. Outcome at 4 years. Indian J Orthop 2018;52:334–8.
28. Brodén B. Roentgen examination of the subtaloid joint in fractures of the calcaneus. Acta Radiol 1949;31:85–8.
29. Hansen ST. Functional reconstruction of the foot and ankle. Philadelphia: Williams & Wilkins; 2000.
30. Sangeorzan BJ, Wagner UA, Harrington RM, et al. Contact characteristics of the subtalar joint: the effect of talar neck misalignment. J Orthop Res 1992;10: 544–51.
31. Zwipp H, Rammelt S. Posttraumatic deformity correction at the foot. Zentralbl Chir 2003;128:218–26 [in German].
32. Rammelt S, Winkler J, Heineck J, et al. Anatomical reconstruction of malunited talus fractures: a prospective study of 10 patients followed for 4 years. Acta Orthop 2005;76:588–96.
33. Rammelt S, Zwipp H. Malunion of the talus. In: Alexander IJ, Bluman EM, Greisberg JK, editors. Advanced reconstruction: foot & ankle 2. Rosemont (IL): The American Academy of Orthopaedic Surgeons (AAOS); 2015. p. 499–508.
34. Monroe MT, Manoli A II. Osteotomy for malunion of a talar neck fracture: a case report. Foot Ankle Int 1999;20:192–5.
35. Asencio G, Rebai M, Bertin R, et al. Pseudarthrosis and non-union of disjunctive talar fractures. Rev Chir Orthop Reparatrice Appar Mot 2000;86:173–80 [in French].
36. Rammelt S, Zwipp H. Secondary correction of talar fractures: asking for trouble? Foot Ankle Int 2012;33(4):359–62.
37. Barg A, Suter T, Nickisch F, et al. Osteotomies of the talar neck for posttraumatic malalignment. Foot Ankle Clin 2016;21(1):77–93.
38. Zwipp H, Rammelt S, Barthel S. Calcaneal fractures–open reduction and internal fixation (ORIF). Injury 2004;35(Suppl 2):SB46–54.
39. Sanders R, Fortin P, DiPasquale T, et al. Operative treatment in 120 displaced intraarticular calcaneal fractures. Results using a prognostic computed tomography scan classification. Clin Orthop Relat Res 1993;290:87–95.
40. Herscovici DJ, Widmaier J, Scaduto JM, et al. Operative treatment of calcaneal fractures in elderly patients. J Bone Joint Surg Am 2005;87(6):1260–4.
41. Gaskill T, Schweitzer K, Nunley J. Comparison of surgical outcomes of intraarticular calcaneal fractures by age. J Bone Joint Surg Am 2012;92(18):2884–9.
42. Benirschke SK, Sangeorzan BJ. Extensive intraarticular fractures of the foot. Surgical management of calcaneal fractures. Clin Orthop 1993;292:128–34.
43. Rammelt S, Zwipp H. Calcaneus fractures: facts, controversies and recent developments. Injury 2004;35:443–61.
44. Sands AK, Rammelt S, Manoli A. Foot compartment syndrome – a clinical review. Fuss Sprungg 2015;13:11–21.
45. Sanders R. Displaced intra-articular fractures of the calcaneus. J Bone Joint Surg Am 2000;82:225–50.
46. Rammelt S, Sangeorzan BJ, Swords MS. Calcaneal fractures – should we or should we not operate? Indian J Orthop 2018;52:220–30.
47. Boack DH, Wichelhaus A, Mittlmeier T, et al. Therapie der dislozierten Calcaneusgelenkfraktur mit der AO-Calcaneusplatte. Chirurg 1998;69(11):1214–23.
48. Brattebo J, Molster AO, Wirsching J. Fractures of the calcaneus: a retrospective study of 115 fractures. Ortho Int 1995;3:117–26.

49. Buckley R, Tough S, McCormack R, et al. Operative compared with nonoperative treatment of displaced intra- articular calcaneal fractures: a prospective, randomized, controlled multicenter trial. J Bone Joint Surg Am 2002;84-A(10):1733–44.

50. Janzen DL, Connell DG, Munk PL, et al. Intraarticular fractures of the calcaneus: value of CT findings in determining prognosis. AJR Am J Roentgenol 1992; 158(6):1271–4.

51. Rammelt S, Barthel S, Biewener A, et al. Calcaneal fractures –open reduction and internal fixation. Zentralbl Chir 2003;128(6):517–28.

52. Rammelt S, Zwipp H, Schneiders W, et al. Severity of injury predicts subsequent function in surgically treated displaced intraarticular calcaneal fractures. Clin Orthop Relat Res 2013;471(9):2885–98.

53. Crosby LA, Fitzgibbons T. Intraarticular calcaneal fractures. Results of closed treatment. Clin Orthop 1993;290:47–54.

54. Mulcahy DM, McCormack DM, Stephens MM. Intraarticular calcaneal fractures: Effect of open reduction and internal fixation on the contact characteristics of the subtalar joint. Foot Ankle Int 1998;19:842–8.

55. Sangeorzan BJ, Ananthakrishnan D, Tencer AF. Contact characteristics of the subtalar joint after a simulated calcaneus fracture. J Orthop Trauma 1995;9: 251–8.

56. Song KS, Kang CH, Min BW, et al. Preoperative and postoperative evaluation of intra-articular fractures of the calcaneus based on computed tomography scanning. J Orthop Trauma 1997;11(6):435–40.

57. Barrick B, Joyce DA, Werner FW, et al. Effect of calcaneus fracture gap without step-off on stress distribution across the subtalar joint. Foot Ankle Int 2017;38: 298–303.

58. Rammelt S, Zwipp H. Fractures of the calcaneus: current treatment strategies. Acta Chir Orthop Traumatol Cech 2014;81:177–96.

59. Gardner MJ, Nork SE, Barei DP, et al. Secondary soft tissue compromise in tongue-type calcaneus fractures. J Orthop Trauma 2008;22:439–45.

60. Swords MP, Penny P. Early fixation of calcaneus fractures. Foot Ankle Clin 2017; 22:93–104.

61. Freeman BJ, Duff S, Allen PE, et al. The extended lateral approach to the hindfoot. Anatomical basis and surgical implications. J Bone Joint Surg Br 1998;80: 139–42.

62. Weber M, Lehmann O, Sagesser D, et al. Limited open reduction and internal fixation of displaced intra-articular fractures of the calcaneum. J Bone Joint Surg Br 2008;90(12):1608–16.

63. Schepers T, Backes M, Dingemans SA, et al. Similar anatomical reduction and lower complication rates with the sinus tarsi approach compared with the extended lateral approach in displaced intra-articular calcaneal fractures. J Orthop Trauma 2017;31:293–8.

64. Hammond AW, Crist BD. Percutaneous treatment of high-risk patients with intra-articular calcaneus fractures: a case series. Injury 2013;44(11):1483–5.

65. Rammelt S, Amlang M, Barthel S, et al. Percutaneous treatment of less severe intraarticular calcaneal fractures. Clin Orthop Relat Res 2010;468(4):983–90.

66. Tornetta P 3rd. The Essex-Lopresti reduction for calcaneal fractures revisited. J Orthop Trauma 1998;12(7):469–73.

67. Rammelt S, Gavlik JM, Barthel S, et al. The value of subtalar arthroscopy in the management of intra-articular calcaneus fractures. Foot Ankle Int 2002;23(10): 906–16.

68. Woon CY, Chong KW, Yeo W, et al. Subtalar arthroscopy and flurosocopy in percutaneous fixation of intra-articular calcaneal fractures: the best of both worlds. J Trauma 2011;71:917–25.

69. Dürr C, Zwipp H, Rammelt S. Fractures of the sustentaculum tali. Oper Orthop Traumatol 2013;25(6):569–78.

70. Sanders R, Vaupel Z, Erdogan M, et al. Operative treatment of displaced intraarticular calcaneal fractures: long-term (10-20 years) results in 108 fractures using a prognostic CT classification. J Orthop Trauma 2014;28(10):551–63.

71. Thordarson DB, Latteier M. Open reduction and internal fixation of calcaneal fractures with a low profile titanium calcaneal perimeter plate. Foot Ankle Int 2003; 24(3):217–21.

72. Richter M, Droste P, Goesling T, et al. Polyaxially-locked plate screws increase stability of fracture fixation in an experimental model of calcaneal fracture. J Bone Joint Surg Br 2006;88(9):1257–63.

73. Illert T, Rammelt S, Drewes T, et al. Stability of locking and non-locking plates in an osteoporotic calcaneal fracture model. Foot Ankle Int 2011;32(3):307–13.

74. Goldzak M, Mittlmeier T, Simon P. Locked nailing for the treatment of displaced articular fractures of the calcaneus: description of a new procedure with calcanail(R). Eur J Orthop Surg Traumatol 2012;22(4):345–9.

75. Zwipp H, Paša L, Žilka L, et al. Introduction of a new locking nail for treatment of intraarticular calcaneal fractures. J Orthop Trauma 2016;30:e88–92.

76. Della Rocca GJ, Nork SE, Barei DP, et al. Fractures of the sustentaculum tali: injury characteristics and surgical technique for reduction. Foot Ankle Int 2009; 30(11):1037–41.

77. Carr J, Hansen S, Benirschke S. Subtalar distraction bone block fusion for late complications of os calcis fractures. Foot Ankle 1998;9(2):81–6.

78. Radnay CS, Clare MP, Sanders RW. Subtalar fusion after displaced intra-articular calcaneal fractures: Does initial operative treatment matter? J Bone Joint Surg Am 2009;91:541–6.

79. Romash MM. Reconstructive osteotomy of the calcaneus with subtalar arthrodesis for malunited calcaneal fractures. Clin Orthop 1993;290(290):157–67.

80. Stephens HM, Sanders R. Calcaneal malunions: results of a prognostic computed tomography classification system. Foot Ankle Int 1996;17(7):395–401.

81. Lui TH. Endoscopic lateral calcaneal ostectomy for calcaneofibular impingement. Arch Orthop Trauma Surg 2007;127(4):265–7.

82. Ketz J, Clare M, Sanders R. Corrective osteotomies for malunited extra-articular calcaneal fractures. Foot Ankle Clin 2016;21(1):135–45.

83. Rammelt S, Grass R, Zwipp H. Joint-preserving osteotomy for malunited intra-articular calcaneal fractures. J Orthop Trauma 2013;27(10):e234–8.

84. Ahn JH, Lee SK, Kim KJ, et al. Subtalar arthroscopic procedures for the treatment of subtalar pathologic conditions: 115 consecutive cases. Orthopedics 2009; 32(12):891.

85. Tasto JP. Arthroscopy of the subtalar joint and arthroscopic subtalar arthrodesis. Instr Course Lect 2006;55:555–64.

86. Brenner P, Zwipp H, Rammelt S. Vascularized double barrel ribs combined with free serratus anterior muscle transfer for homologous restoration of the hindfoot after calcanectomy. J Trauma 2000;49(2):331–5.

Cavus Foot
Deciding Between Osteotomy and Arthrodesis

Mark S. Myerson, MD[a], C. Lucas Myerson, BA[b],*

KEYWORDS

- Cavus foot • Coleman block test • Moderate deformity
- Midfoot osteotomy-arthrodesis • Soft tissue balancing

KEY POINTS

- Most mistakes in surgical decision-making occur when trying to correct moderate cavus deformity.
- The Coleman block test may not be sufficient for predicting the ability of an osteotomy-based procedure to correct deformity.
- Moderate deformity is characterized by an increased cavus of the midfoot and increased supination laterally.
- The key to the treatment of moderate deformity is the midfoot osteotomy or arthrodesis.

INTRODUCTION

There are many cavus feet in which the decision-making for correction is easy. This applies in particular to those rigid deformities in which just by looking at the foot one is able to determine that a procedure combining various osteotomies and tendon transfers will not be sufficient for treatment (**Fig. 1**).[1]

It is the foot that has a mild to moderate cavus deformity that creates the dilemma. This article addresses these deformities and provides an outline for decision-making with respect to correction (**Fig. 2**).

Perhaps the first issue that one has to address is the flexibility of the foot. To determine flexibility of the hindfoot and forefoot, the Coleman block test is frequently used (**Fig. 3**).[2–5] This test is acceptable appreciate the mobility of the hindfoot and, in particular, the subtalar joint.[6] This test, however, should not guide one to a specific treatment.

More important than a specific test such as the Coleman block examination is the examination of the foot. In particular, we find that it is more useful to get a feel for hindfoot flexibility by manipulating the subtalar joint with the foot in slight plantarflexion

The authors have nothing to disclose.
[a] Steps2Walk, 1209 Harbor Island Walk, Baltimore, MD 21230, USA; [b] Tulane University School of Medicine, 1430 Tulane Avenue, New Orleans, LA 70112, USA
* Corresponding author.
E-mail address: lucasmyerson@gmail.com

Foot Ankle Clin N Am 24 (2019) 347–360
https://doi.org/10.1016/j.fcl.2019.02.007
1083-7515/19/© 2019 Elsevier Inc. All rights reserved.

foot.theclinics.com

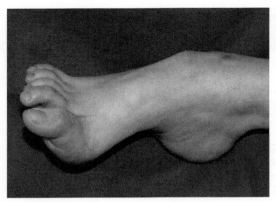

Fig. 1. There are deformities that, just by looking at the foot, one is able to determine that a procedure combining various osteotomies and tendon transfers will not be sufficient for treatment.

(**Fig. 4**). In the more flexible cavus foot, this manipulation gives one a good sense of how everting the hindfoot into valgus influences forefoot position. In the flexible foot, the more subtalar mobility that is present, the more the first metatarsal will be forced into equinus with this maneuver.

The authors prefer not to rely on the Coleman block test to determine the type of surgery to be performed. In a recent unpublished study of more than 470 cavus foot surgeries, 172 subjects were identified who had undergone a surgery with 1 or more osteotomies in conjunction with various tendon transfers (Maccario C, Kaplan J, Myerson M. Failure of the Coleman block test to adequately predict deformity correction for the mild to moderate cavus foot, unpublished data, 2017). No arthrodesis of the midfoot or hindfoot was performed in this group of subjects. The radiographs of these 172 subjects were subsequently examined and only 38% had satisfactory correction of the deformity. In the remaining subjects, although there was some improvement in the alignment, there were many residual radiographic findings of deformity. These included a subtalar joint that remained in varus, or a midfoot

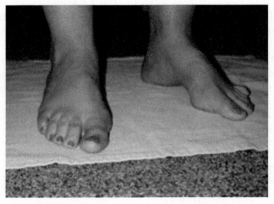

Fig. 2. A mild to moderate deformity in which decision-making becomes more difficult with respect to surgical correction.

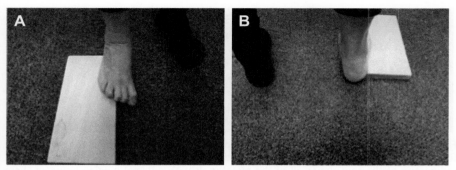

Fig. 3. To perform the Coleman block test, (A) the lateral foot is placed on the block and the first metatarsal is allowed to come to the ground. (B) Some correction of heel varus to neutral is achieved, suggesting that the hindfoot is flexible.

that was either supinated or remained slightly adducted. The supination of the midfoot was particularly noticeable by analyzing the ratio of the position of the fifth metatarsal and the medial cuneiform to the floor preoperatively and postoperatively. In many of these subjects, this ratio was not corrected postoperatively (**Fig. 5**).

There are simple measurements that one can rely on to analyze the position of the first metatarsal to the fifth metatarsal, both with respect to the declination of the first metatarsal and the height of the fifth metatarsal from the floor. Regardless of the degree of deformity or the type of surgery performed, on the lateral view, the height of the medial cuneiform to the floor should decrease postoperatively. In addition, the position and height of the fifth metatarsal from the floor should increase postoperatively.

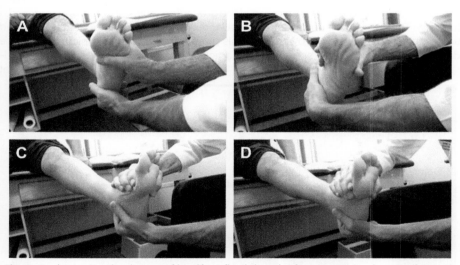

Fig. 4. To determine the degree of hindfoot flexibility, the foot is examined manually. Hindfoot flexibility can be appreciated by placing the foot in slight plantarflexion and then manipulating the subtalar joint. (A, B) A flexible foot with good subtalar motion. The valgus stress on the hindfoot forces the first metatarsals into equinus. (C, D) Manipulation of the hindfoot can influence forefoot position.

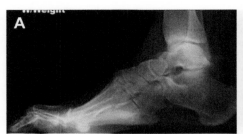
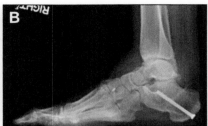

Fig. 5. A supination-type deformity is accompanied by midfoot rotation that results in a fifth metatarsal that is closer to the floor than the medial cuneiform. (A) Preoperative lateral radiograph of the foot shows all of the metatarsals with minimal overlap between them (ie, stacking of the metatarsals). (B) Postoperative radiograph in which derotation of the midfoot has been achieved. The ratio of the distance of the fifth metatarsal and the medial cuneiform to the floor has improved but not completely corrected because the fifth metatarsal is still too close to the ground.

On the anteroposterior view of the foot, the adduction or varus of the forefoot relative to the hindfoot should improve with a change, not only in the coverage of the talonavicular (TN) joint but also in the alignment of the talus with respect to the first metatarsal (**Fig. 6**).

In the group of 172 subjects previously described, the Coleman block test was routinely used. Based on this test, it was assumed preoperatively that these feet were flexible enough that a surgery could be performed that did not include arthrodesis. It was concluded, however, that for most subjects in the study group, the Coleman block test was not sufficient to predict the ability of an osteotomy-based procedure to correct the deformity. Although this study focused on the radiographic correction of the procedure, one might be also be able to extrapolate from these radiographic results the functional outcomes of the procedure. This has to do with form and function. That is to say, if correction of the alignment (the form) is imperfect, the function of the foot may not improve much. This does not always hold clinically but that discussion is beyond the scope of this article. The authors think that the most

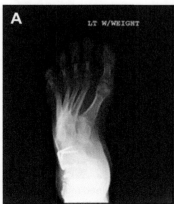
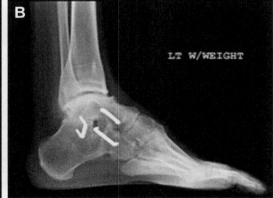

Fig. 6. A severe recurrent deformity after a failed triple arthrodesis, which demonstrates persistent forefoot adductovarus deformity. (A,B) The coverage of the TN joint is poor and alignment of the talus is inadequate with respect to the first metatarsal.

important step in the evaluation of the cavus foot is identifying the deforming forces involved. Invariably the peroneus longus muscle will be stronger than the anterior tibial muscle and the posterior tibial muscle will be stronger than the peroneus brevis muscle.[7] Additionally, a variable degree of contracture of the gastrocnemius and soleus muscles is present.

DECISION-MAKING

A principle of deformity correction and, in particular, the cavus foot, is to perform the osteotomy at the apex of the deformity.[6] In the previously noted series of 470 cavus foot surgery procedures, there were 172 subjects who had flexible deformities. For these flexible deformities, surgery was performed with 1 or more osteotomies. At that time, these generally included the first metatarsal and the calcaneus. Although the first metatarsal frequently underwent an osteotomy, it is essential to recognize that the apex of the cavus deformity is never at or in the first metatarsal.[8] This is structurally impossible. The apex of the deformity is always proximal to the base of the first metatarsal, either at the first tarsometatarsal (TMT) joint, the cuneiform, the naviculo-cuneiform (NC), or the TN joint.

Why then is a dorsiflexion osteotomy of the first metatarsal so frequently performed? Although elevating the metatarsal head with this osteotomy may correct the distal overload of the first metatarsal, it is technically incorrect and can lead to a boat-shaped deformity of the forefoot[2] (**Fig. 7**). It is the authors' preference, therefore, to perform the osteotomy or arthrodesis directly at the apex of the deformity, which will either be the first TMT joint, the medial cuneiform, the NC joint, or the TN joint, as previously described. A first metatarsal osteotomy should be used only for convenience purposes for subtle mild deformities.

WHAT IS A FLEXIBLE AND MILD DEFORMITY?

A flexible and mild deformity is difficult to quantify but it implies that the subtalar joint is easily correctable to neutral, there is minimal forefoot equinus deformity, and there is absence of an adductovarus deformity.[1] In addition, there is only mild supination of the midfoot. For the flexible foot associated with the minor deformity, we perform a combination of a plantar fascia release, a calcaneal osteotomy, a transfer of the peroneus longus to brevis, and then whatever else is necessary to complete the correction.[9-11] Additional procedures may include a first metatarsal osteotomy, an arthrodesis of the first TMT joint, or a closing wedge osteotomy of the medial cuneiform.[12,13] An associated equinus deformity is often present, which can be corrected with either a percutaneous Achilles lengthening or a gastrocnemius recession. The calcaneus osteotomy

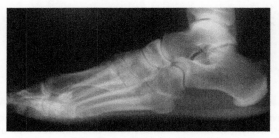

Fig. 7. Dorsiflexion osteotomy of the first metatarsal. There is boat-shaped deformity of the forefoot produced secondary to elevation of the first metatarsal head.

is a very utilitarian procedure to correct the cavus foot and, depending on the magnitude of the deformity, is always required in some form. For instance, there are times when a biplanar calcaneus osteotomy is added to a subtalar arthrodesis to correct a very severe hindfoot varus deformity.

WHAT IS A MODERATE DEFORMITY?

This type of deformity is characterized by an increased cavus of the midfoot, as well as increased supination laterally, which creates a much greater load, not only under the fifth metatarsal head but also along the entire length of the fifth metatarsal. If adductovarus is present, it is typically mild. For that reason, a transfer of the posterior tibial tendon (PTT) is unusual in these cases unless the cavus is caused by Charcot-Marie-Tooth (CMT) disease.[14,15] CMT may be associated with a drop foot, which could be managed with transfer of the PTT through the interosseous membrane to the dorsocentral midfoot.[4] For the correction of moderate deformity, the same sequence of procedures used for mild deformity is performed. These procedures alone will not be sufficient to correct the deformity of the midfoot. The key to the treatment of moderate deformity is the midfoot osteotomy or arthrodesis.

THE MIDFOOT OSTEOTOMY-ARTHRODESIS

The authors use this procedure frequently in cases of mild to moderate cavus deformity in which some flexibility in the foot remains but a more extensive hindfoot arthrodesis is not necessary.[5] The indication for this procedure is a moderate cavus deformity associated with a varus deformity of the heel, a plantarflexed first metatarsal, and an apex of the deformity in the midfoot. As previously mentioned, the decision as to the location of the procedure for all cavus foot correction is based on the apex of the deformity.[16] This will vary in some cases and may even be associated with multiple apices (**Fig. 8**).

Note that if the midfoot osteotomy-arthrodesis is not performed at the apex of the deformity, one can expect some but not complete improvement in the alignment (**Fig. 9**). In cases of multiple apices, a triple arthrodesis is commonly performed. In these cases, a second procedure must be performed to correct the additional, more distal apex, which will not correct with the hindfoot arthrodesis. This second apex is generally in the midfoot, either at the first TMT joint or a little more proximally at the cuneiform. The midfoot osteotomy-arthrodesis is always performed at the apex

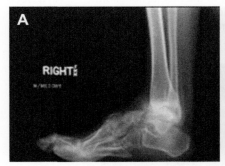
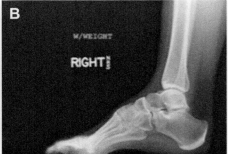

Fig. 8. These 2 cavus feet demonstrate how important it is to determine the apex of the deformity preoperatively. (*A*) Severe hindfoot varus and midfoot supination but an apex at the level of the NC joint. (*B*) A more global cavus forefoot deformity is present without rotation of the midfoot and an apex more proximally at the TN joint.

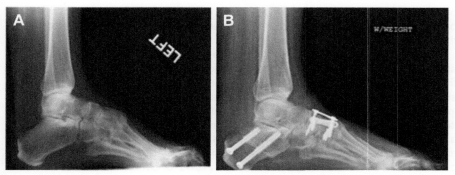

Fig. 9. The midfoot osteotomy-arthrodesis is demonstrated. (*A*) The apex preoperatively is located more distally at the TMT joint. (*B*) This was not completely corrected with the procedure because there is a persistent mild deformity at the TMT joint even though the rotation of the midfoot is improved.

of the deformity, which may correspond to the navicular or the cuneiforms or, rarely, slightly more anteriorly at the TMT joints. Therefore, a combination of an arthrodesis, usually of the NC joints, and an osteotomy of the cuneiform is performed.

If the apex is slightly more anterior than the NC joints, then an osteotomy can be performed across the entire midfoot with the removal of a biplanar, dorsomedially based wedge.[16] This wedge is started on the dorsal surface of the medial cuneiform and then the wedge is removed from medial to lateral entering the cuboid. A wedge is never removed from the cuboid but, invariably, the cuboid should be cut through the midsection. This allows one to rotate and elevate the cuboid, which corrects the midfoot supination deformity. It is rare that wedge correction can be obtained with a single bone cut. The declination of the first metatarsal is always more depressed than the fifth, so a biplanar wedge must be made. When a biplanar wedge is performed, more bone is removed from the dorsal than from the lateral midfoot (**Fig. 10**). It is very important to understand that one cannot remove a medially based wedge

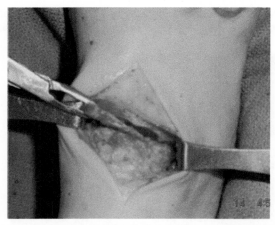

Fig. 10. The osteotomy or osteotomy-arthrodesis is performed at the apex of the deformity, in this case through the cuneiforms and cuboid. No bone is removed from the cuboid, and the wedge is removed dorsomedially.

because this will cause or worsen any adductus deformity. The wedge is, therefore, based dorsally toward the middle and medial cuneiform but tapered laterally into the cuboid where no wedge is removed.

The surgical approach includes an extensile incision made in the midline of the foot and extends from the ankle joint distally through the midfoot. The entire midfoot from the medial cuneiform to the cuboid must be visualized, and a shorter incision can cause skin necrosis or dehiscence secondary to excessive retraction. For that reason, we use a longer incision for our approach. The superficial and deep peroneal nerves are retracted laterally and medially, and then the soft tissue is elevated with subperiosteal dissection and retracted medially. One will often note that the muscle of the extensor hallucis brevis appears a little white or pink as a result of intrinsic muscle atrophy. This makes it easier to cut the extensor hallucis brevis tendon, which allows for better exposure of the dorso-medial midfoot. The entire central aspect of the midfoot is then stripped using a wide curved periosteal elevator. We like to use electrocautery to mark out the proposed osteotomy (**Fig. 11**), which should be done under fluoroscopic guidance to delineate the apex of the deformity medially and center of the cuboid laterally.

The plane of correction depends entirely on the shape of the foot. If the cavus is un-accompanied by additional midfoot deformity, an osteotomy or arthrodesis of the NC or TMT joint will suffice. In those cases, an osteotomy will consist of a wedge that begins medially and is based on the dorsal surface.

On the other hand, there may be additional deformity, such as adduction or supination, of the midfoot. With a supination-type deformity there is rotation of the midfoot such that the fifth metatarsal is lower and closer to the floor than the medial cuneiform. This can always be seen on the radiograph with stacking of the metatarsals, in which all of the metatarsals are visible on a lateral view of the foot with minimal overlap.[4] In that situation, a cut can be made that tapers to the lateral side of the midfoot and ends in the cuboid. Proper alignment of the midfoot is then achieved by elevating the lateral side of the foot through rotation of the cuboid. In addition, the distal aspect of the cuboid must be pushed dorsally to correct the deformity.

It is common that one will have to remove a large wedge from the dorsal medial cuneiform when an osteotomy is performed. The base of the osteotomy is dorsal, and the cut will then be varied to some extent in accordance with the shape of the foot. As the osteotomy moves further laterally, less bone is resected, and the correction is obtained more by dorsal elevation and rotation of the lateral border of the foot than through wedge correction (**Fig. 12**). It is difficult to predict the size of the wedge

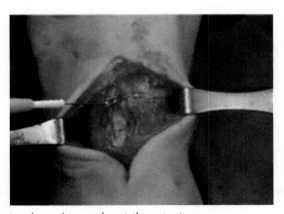

Fig. 11. Electrocautery is used to mark out the osteotomy.

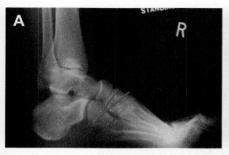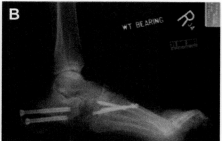

Fig. 12. (*A*) A wedge is planned through the apex of the deformity at the level of the NC joints and the cuboid. (*B*) The midfoot was elevated and rotated to gain more satisfactory correction of the forefoot cavus.

and the extent of rotation and, although preoperative planning will determine the location of the bone cut, most of the fine-tuning is done intraoperatively. A saw is used to perform the osteotomy or bone removal from the joint, which we find is far more accurate than using an osteotome. If the dorsal position of the apex is in the NC joint, the medial exit point usually is at the base of the medial cuneiform and, to have adequate exposure, the anterior tibial tendon attachment must be reflected and retracted medially. The wedge cut is then shaped such that the medial limb is approximately 8 mm at a 15-degree to 20-degree angle to the dorsal plane of the midfoot.

Bone is resected only dorsally because any medial wedge will adduct the midfoot, which is never desirable. If a cavus deformity only of the midfoot is present, then the dorsal base of the osteotomy extends from the center of the foot medially at much the same distance as that between the osteotomy limbs. The first lateral osteotomy cut is made extending toward the cuboid from the middle or lateral cuneiform, and then the second osteotomy cut is made at a much smaller angle so that the apex is in the cuboid without removing much of the cuboid at all. The lateral correction is accomplished by translating the distal cuboid dorsally, and then rotating it slightly, which will elevate the base of the fifth metatarsal. After the wedges have been resected, the forefoot is then dorsiflexed until good contact between the dorsal bone surfaces is achieved. The advantage of this osteotomy is that further contouring can be performed, just as with any wedge osteotomy, until sufficient bone has been removed and the forefoot position relative to the hindfoot has been corrected. Often, after the wedge is removed, the 2 ends of the bone do not appose and it is necessary to elevate the distal part of the foot more dorsally to gain more correction of the forefoot cavus (**Fig. 13**).

It is difficult to fix this type of osteotomy with plates or screws. Occasionally, staples can be used, particularly if an arthrodesis is performed; however, if an osteotomy of the cuneiforms is performed, then the staples will always be too large and cross into 1 of the adjacent joints. Use of staples is, therefore, only possible if adequate bone is present on both sides of the osteotomy or arthrodesis, which is not usually the case. Crossing screws can be used but these traverse joints that have not been included in the osteotomy or arthrodesis. Generally, we only use screws when an arthrodesis of the midfoot is performed. Our preferred method of fixation is with pins. The use of 2-mm or 2.5-mm pins in this location is much easier because of the plane of the osteotomy or arthrodesis and the small bone segments between each articulation. Frequently, therefore, we insert large crossed pins from the medial and lateral portion of the foot, from distal to proximal, and then remove them at

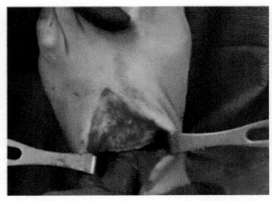

Fig. 13. To elevate the cuboid, an osteotome inserted into the osteotomy to elevate cuboid and rotate the midfoot.

6 weeks in children and 8 weeks in adults after ambulation in a cast or boot begins. Healing of these osteotomies, as well as the midfoot arthrodesis, is generally quite predictable.

SOFT TISSUE BALANCE AND TENDON TRANSFER

A plantar fascia release invariably needs to be performed regardless of the magnitude of the deformity.[12] The primary deformity begins as a result of muscle imbalance between the PTT and the peroneus brevis, which causes the hindfoot varus deformity and, with progression, adductovarus of the midfoot.

As the heel moves into varus, the first metatarsal has to compensate for the hindfoot position. To maintain the forefoot in a plantigrade position, the first metatarsal drops into equinus. This equinus position of the first metatarsal is perpetuated and aggravated by contracture of the plantar fascia and, in cases in which there is weakness of the anterior tibial muscle such as that associated with CMT, the equinus of the first metatarsal is worsened. With increasing contracture of the plantar fascia and, in particular, as a result of atrophy of the intrinsic muscles of the foot, the forefoot deformity worsens.

The plantar fascia release is usually the first procedure that we perform because the calcaneus osteotomy is difficult to perform correctly if the plantar fascia is contracted.[16] The authors recommend performing the fascia release through a medial longitudinal incision adjacent to the heel, at the junction of the dorsal and plantar skin. Unfortunately, some patients may be left with a small patch of numbness on the medial aspect of the heel pad from this incision, and the potential for this outcome must be explained to patients preoperatively. The incision is made over a 2-cm length it must be just dorsal to the heel pad above the origin of the fascia. The fascia is initially cut under direct visualization, immediately anterior to the calcaneus, using scissors advanced from medial to lateral. After the scissors have been introduced, the release can be completed blindly through palpation. The scissors are advanced without a cutting motion until both the medial and lateral bands are completely released. For a severe deformity in which cavo-adductovarus is present, the fascia of the abductor hallucis tendon may also require a release. For some of these severe deformities, the intrinsic muscles must be stripped off the calcaneus completely, in addition to the fascia release.

PERONEUS LONGUS TO BREVIS TRANSFER

The peroneus longus-to-brevis tendon transfer is an essential procedure for all types of cavus deformity. We use this transfer for almost all types of deformities, including more mild and flexible feet in which there seems to be an imbalance between the strength of the peroneal muscles.[3] Certainly, in moderate and severe deformity, this procedure is essential because the transfer augments the weak peroneus brevis muscle and decreases the force on plantarflexion of the first metatarsal.[7] The procedure will have much more impact on the flexible foot than the rigid foot. In advanced cases of very rigid cavus deformities, the authors do not expect the impact of the transfer to be as significant, particularly if a triple and midfoot arthrodesis is performed. Although the longus can be cut and then transferred into the brevis, we prefer to suture both tendons together before cutting the longus. In so doing, we ensure that the tension on the transfer is correct, which is difficult to obtain if the longus is cut first[3] (**Fig. 14**).

POSTERIOR TIBIAL TENDON TRANSFER

As previously stated, there is always muscle imbalance in the cavus foot. The peroneus longus muscle will be stronger than the anterior tibial muscle, and the posterior tibial muscle will be stronger than the peroneus brevis muscle. For the mild to moderate deformities, we always include a peroneus longus to peroneus brevis transfer. A PTT transfer is performed, in particular to correct a paralytic cavovarus deformity, which includes a foot drop.[9] The main advantage of the PTT transfer is to improve dorsiflexion when paralysis is present but, more importantly, it simultaneously removes the deforming force of the posterior tibial muscle in severe cases of cavoadductovarus. The PTT is a nonphasic tendon transfer, so if there is no adductovarus and the extensor hallucis longus and extensor digitorum longus are functioning, then these may be used preferentially for the tendon transfer to augment dorsiflexion.[7]

CALCANEUS OSTEOTOMY

After the fascia has been cut, we proceed laterally to the calcaneus osteotomy, which is performed in every cavus foot regardless of the magnitude of deformity. The incision for the calcaneus osteotomy varies according to the type of procedure performed.[9] If an osteotomy alone is performed, then a shorter incision is made directly inferior to the

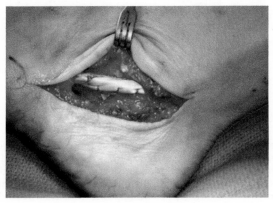

Fig. 14. Tendon transfer of peroneus longus to peroneus brevis To ensure proper tension on the tendon transfer, both tendons are sutured together before trimming peroneus longus.

peroneal tendons. Often, however, the calcaneus osteotomy needs to be performed with additional lateral procedures, including repair of the peroneal tendon, reconstruction of the lateral ankle for instability, or a peroneus longus to brevis tendon transfer.[3] For these cases, the incision is simply extended posteriorly along the axis of the peroneal tendons behind the fibula. The technical details of this osteotomy are well-described in the paper (See Federico Giuseppe Usuelli and Luigi Manzi's article, "Inframalleolar Varus Deformity: Role of Calcaneal Osteotomies," in this issue) and will not be further discussed here.

SUMMARY

As previously noted, it is easy to distinguish between a mild and a severe cavus deformity. These do not seem to present a problem as far as deciding on a treatment is concerned. The difficulty lies in the approach to more moderate deformity in which the foot appears to be correctible on a Coleman block test, the hindfoot is flexible on examination, and one tries to avoid an arthrodesis. The authors think this is when most

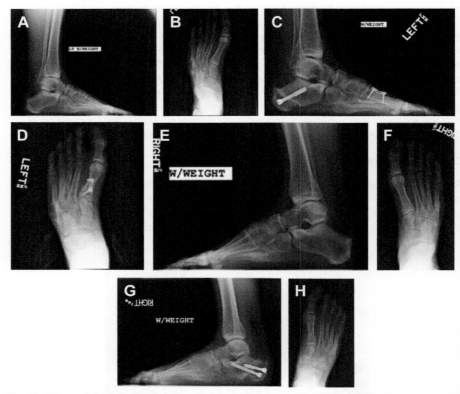

Fig. 15. Bilateral flexible cavus deformity in an adolescent. (*A–D*) The left foot was managed first with a calcaneus and first metatarsal osteotomy, a plantar fascia release, and a transfer of longus to the brevis. The foot is not adequately corrected postoperatively. (*C, D*) Varus deformity of the subtalar joint persists, and there is overload of the fifth metatarsal secondary to supination of the midfoot. (*E, F*) The opposite foot was treated with a midfoot osteotomy-arthrodesis. (*G, H*) Note the satisfactory correction of the hindfoot varus and derotation of the midfoot.

mistakes are made in decision-making. It is difficult to determine whether a foot is flexible and, in our experience, we undertreated many of these flexible feet. An example is an adolescent with bilateral flexible cavus deformity. The first foot operated on was done in what most surgeons would consider a traditional procedure, with a calcaneus and first metatarsal osteotomy, a plantar fascia release, and a transfer of longus to the brevis. The foot was not adequately corrected postoperatively (**Fig. 15**). The subtalar joint remained in varus, and there was severe persistent supination of the midfoot with overload of the fifth metatarsal clearly evident. So, why did this happen? We were probably misled by the flexibility of the hindfoot. We failed to appreciate the severity of the deformity and this led to undertreatment. In retrospect, there was probably too much midfoot supination deformity to expect that this would correct with a simpler osteotomy-based procedure. Although there was symptomatic improvement postoperatively, the authors thought it would be preferable to change the surgical approach in the opposite foot, and a midfoot osteotomy-arthrodesis was performed. It was possible to correct the foot at the apex of the deformity and, in particular, to rotate and elevate the cuboid through the osteotomy. The postoperative radiograph following surgery demonstrated very good correction of the hindfoot, the subtalar joint included, as well as the midfoot, which is now plantigrade.

REFERENCES

1. Olney B. Treatment of the cavus foot. Deformity in the pediatric patient with Charcot-Marie-Tooth. Foot Ankle Clin 2000;5:305–15.

2. Deben SE, Pomeroy GC. Subtle cavus foot: diagnosis and management. J Am Acad Orthop Surg 2014;22(8):512–20.

3. Krause FG, Wing KJ, Younger AS. Neuromuscular issues in cavovarus foot. Foot Ankle Clin 2008;13:243–58, vi.

4. Maynou C, Szymanski C, Thiounn A. The adult cavus foot. EFORT Open Rev 2017;2(5):221–9.

5. Nogueira MP, Farcetta F, Zuccon A. Cavus foot. Foot Ankle Clin 2015;20(4):645–56.

6. Zide JR, Myerson MS. Arthrodesis for the cavus foot: when, where, and how? Foot Ankle Clin 2013;18(4):755–67.

7. Huber M. What is the role of tendon transfer in the cavus foot? Foot Ankle Clin 2013;(4):689–95.

8. Aminian A, Sangeorzan BJ. The anatomy of cavus foot deformity. Foot Ankle Clin 2008;13:191–8, v.

9. Jung HG, Park JT, Lee SH. Joint-sparing correction for idiopathic cavus foot: correlation of clinical and radiographic results. Foot Ankle Clin 2013;18(4):659–71.

10. Sammarco GJ, Taylor R. Combined calcaneal and metatarsal osteotomies for the treatment of cavus foot. Foot Ankle Clin 2001;6:533–43, vii.

11. VanValkenburg S, Hsu RY, Palmer DS, et al. Neurologic deficit associated with lateralizing calcaneal osteotomy for cavovarus foot correction. Foot Ankle Int 2016;37(10):1106–12.

12. Ward CM, Dolan LA, Bennett DL, et al. Long-term results of reconstruction for treatment of a flexible cavovarus foot in Charcot-Marie-Tooth disease. J Bone Joint Surg Am 2008;90:2631–42.

13. Wulker N, Hurschler C. Cavus foot correction in adults by dorsal closing wedge osteotomy. Foot Ankle Int 2002;23:344–7.

14. Dreher T, Wolf SI, Heitzmann D, et al. Tibialis posterior tendon transfer corrects the foot drop component of cavovarus foot deformity in Charcot-Marie-Tooth disease. J Bone Joint Surg Am 2014;96(6):456–62.
15. Laurá M, Singh D, Ramdharry G, et al. Prevalence and orthopedic management of foot and ankle deformities in Charcot–Marie–Tooth disease. Muscle Nerve 2018;57(2):255–9.
16. Myerson MS, Kadakia AR. Cavus foot correction. In: Reconstructive foot and ankle surgery. Management of complications. 3rd edition. Philadelphia: Elsevier; 2019. p. 141–54.

Failure of Surgical Treatment in Patients with Cavovarus Deformity
Why Does This Happen and How Do We Approach Treatment?

Shuyuan Li, MD, PhD*, Mark S. Myerson, MD

KEYWORDS

- Cavus foot • Surgery • Arthrodesis • Osteotomy • Apex of the deformity
- Muscle imbalance • Mutiplanar deformity

KEY POINTS

- There is not as much role for the Coleman block test to determine flexibility of the foot, and this has led to many failures where we believed the foot to be flexible, and indeed an osteotomy was insufficient treatment.
- The apex in the sagittal plane is either in the midfoot or the hindfoot and determines the location as well as the type of the procedure that should be performed.
- The typical tendon transfer for the cavus foot is to use the posterior tibial tendon and place it in a position that is beneficial for the foot and ankle, particularly with respect to regaining some dorsiflexion power. There is a multiplanar deformity and the procedures are not performed at multiple levels (apices).
- An adductovarus deformity of the midfoot is a more severe variant of the cavus foot and can be an adductus of the midfoot associated with varus of the hindfoot or adductus associated with hindfoot varus and forefoot cavus as well as equinus.
- Beware of the patient with a significant callosity under the base of the fifth metatarsal. This is always associated with a severe hindfoot varus and supination of the midfoot and also at times associated with adduction of the midfoot.

INTRODUCTION

Published results of the triple arthrodesis for cavus foot deformity demonstrate variable outcomes. There is a range of procedures available for correction of deformity, and the mainstay of correction for severe deformity is an arthrodesis of some form,

The authors have nothing to disclose.
Steps2Walk, 1209 Harbor Island Walk, Baltimore, MD 21230, USA
* Corresponding author.
E-mail address: drshuyuanli@gmail.com

Foot Ankle Clin N Am 24 (2019) 361–370
https://doi.org/10.1016/j.fcl.2019.02.008
1083-7515/19/© 2019 Elsevier Inc. All rights reserved.

generally including the hindfoot. This article discusses more severe deformities and focus on the causes of deformity, without a discussion of the more minor and moderate deformities. It is a common error to assume that cavus feet are similar. Almost every cavus foot that the authors treat is slightly different from the next.

A RIGID AND NOT A FLEXIBLE DEFORMITY IS PRESENT

Please see Mark S. Myerson and C. Lucas Myerson's article, "Cavus Foot: Deciding Between Osteotomy and Arthrodesis," in this issue for a more extensive discussion on this topic.[1–4] Suffice it to state that although it is easy to determine the presence of severe deformity, those that are mild and moderate frequently lead to difficulties with decision making and recurrent deformity.[5] This complication is highlighted in **Fig. 1**, a case of a 31-year-old man who presented with recurrent deformity after attempted correction with a calcaneus and first metatarsal osteotomy. The subtalar joint remains in varus, the midfoot is supinated, there is overload of the fifth metatarsal, and the hindfoot is in varus alignment (see **Fig. 1**).

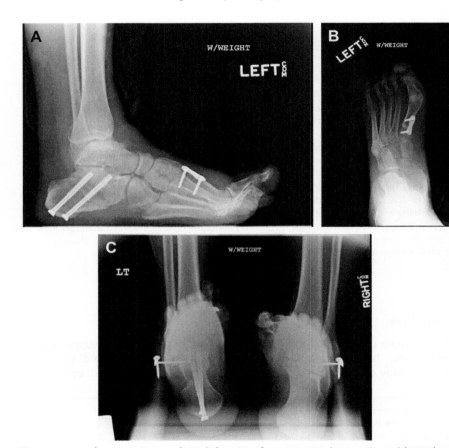

Fig. 1. A case of recurrent cavus foot deformity after attempted correction with a calcaneus and first metatarsal osteotomy. Note the subtalar joint remains in varus on the lateral view (*A*), the midfoot is supinated on both lateral and AP views (*A, B*), there is overload of the fifth metatarsal (*A*), and the hindfoot is still in varus alignment (*C*).

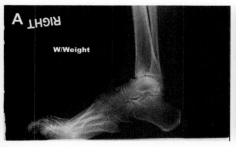
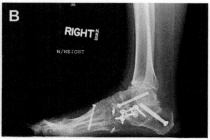

Fig. 2. A case of recurrent cavus foot deformity after a first metatarsal osteotomy and a double arhtrodesis in the hindfoot. Note that the apex of the midfoot cavus was at the level of the first TMT joint before the surgery (*A*), yet a first metatarsal osteotomy was performed (*B*), leading to a dorsiflexion malunion of the metatarsal.

THE CORRECTION IS NOT PERFORMED AT THE APEX OF THE DEFORMITY

The apex in the sagittal plane is either in the midfoot or the hindfoot and determines the location and type of the procedure that should be performed. The medial column of the foot is always more plantarflexed than the lateral column, but the lateral column tends to be more fixed and rotated. Thus, when correcting the plantarflexion of the first ray, rotational malalignment also must be addressed or else the foot is left in a supinated position with continued overload of the lateral column.

Occasionally, the apex of the deformity is more distal, that is, at the level of the tarsometatarsal joint (TMT), and an arthrodesis of this joint, in particular the first TMT joint, should be performed and not a first metatarsal osteotomy (**Fig. 2**). In such a situation like the case in **Fig. 2**, a first metatarsal osteotomy instead of a first TMT joint arthrodesis was performed, leading to a dorsiflexion malunion of the first metatarsal. Jahss[6] described a truncated wedge arthrodesis of the entire TMT joint for this type of deformity, but a global cavus at the level of the TMT joints is rare. The TMT truncated wedge arthrodesis procedure is technically easy to perform, but the arthrodesis must be balanced, removing more bone from the first TMT joint and then less at the second and third. It is extremely rare that an arthrodesis of the fourth and fifth metatarsal joints is performed, unless a very severe midfoot cavus is present. Instead, the arthrodesis of the medial 3 joints is performed in conjunction with an osteotomy of the cuboid in order to elevate and then rotate the lateral foot and correct the overload on the fifth metatarsal. It is rare that a wedge needs to be removed from the cuboid metatarsal articulation. Even if the apex is at the TMT, the rest of the foot cannot be ignored, and complete correction must be performed. In the case illustrated, the medial apex does seem to be at the first TMT joint preoperatively, but the rest of the deformity was not taken into consideration during the correction. The midfoot remains significantly rotated with the fifth metatarsal close to the floor, and although there has been some correction at the first TMT joint, there is persistent deformity present (**Fig. 3**). A different error was noted in a patient with a cavus foot but mostly as a result of a calcaneus deformity, with a very high pitch angle of the calcaneus associated with arthritis of the hindfoot and a global cavus of the forefoot with no midfoot rotational deformity. Although the triple arthrodesis was a logical procedure to perform, this should have been corrected in conjunction with a calcaneus osteotomy, shifting the tuberosity cephalad to decrease the pitch angle. This is technically easy to perform using the same screw for the osteotomy as the subtalar arthrodesis (**Fig. 4**).[7,8]

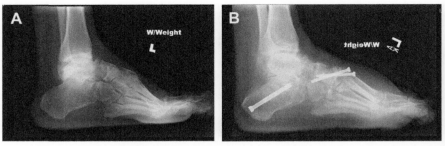

Fig. 3. A case of cavus foot deformity (*A*). The deformity recurred after correction focusing only on the first TMT joint (*B*), whereas the rest of the midfoot deformity was neglected. Note that the midfoot remains significantly rotated with the fifth metatarsal close to the floor.

MUSCLE IMBALANCE IS PRESENT AND A TENDON TRANSFER IS NOT PERFORMED

In the typical cavovarus foot, the deforming forces are the tibialis posterior and the peroneus longus, which overpower the peroneus brevis and tibialis anterior, which leads to the varus hindfoot and pronated and plantarflexed medial column. The typical tendon transfer for the cavus foot is to use the posterior tibial tendon (PTT) and place it in a position that is beneficial for the foot and ankle, particularly with respect to

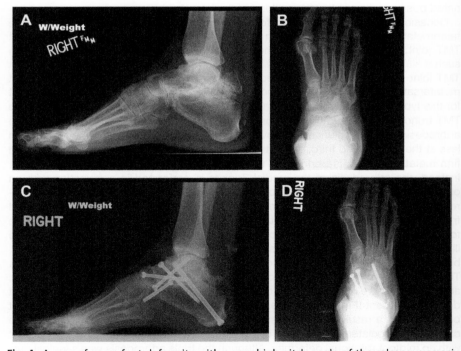

Fig. 4. A case of cavus foot deformity with a very high pitch angle of the calcaneus associated with arthritis of the hindfoot (*A, B*). A triple arthrodesis had been done (*C, D*), but the deformity recurred. Note the uncorrected high pitch angle (*C*), which should be addressed with adding a calcneus osteotomy to the triple arthrodesis, shifting the tuberosity cephalad to decrease the pitch angle.

regaining some dorsiflexion power. Muscle power of any commonly transferred tendon in the cavus foot, however, in particular the posterior tibial, is variable. It must be recognized that the benefit of a tendon transfer not only is the dynamic function that it exerts on the foot but also, more importantly, the removal of the force of that muscle, regardless of its power. When the muscle is weak, surgeons often do not use it as a tendon transfer, believing it too weak for the transfer. This, however, creates a failure because there is always some power left in the muscle that overcomes its antagonist and gradually leads to recurrence of deformity. Cavovarus deformities tend to be both dynamic and progressive and only a well-balanced foot is stable over time. Soft tissue balancing contributes to the long-term success of the arthrodesis, because it removes the major deforming forces going forward.[9–11]

Soft tissue balancing, by means of tendon transfers and release of the plantar fascia and occasionally the abductor fascia, must be included in the correction. If the deformity is absolutely rigid with no function of the posterior tibial muscle present, then a tenotomy of the tendon can be performed to assist with the revision correction (**Fig. 5**). There are numerous reports of failure, specifically of triple arthrodesis, but the authors believe this is the result of incomplete correction or, more importantly, where muscle balance of the foot was not obtained. Muscle balance is essential to the successful outcome of correction of the cavus foot. Considering the dynamic nature of these deformities, and an arthrodesis, even a triple arthrodesis, cannot maintain correction of the deformity, because these tendons insert distal to the level of the arthrodesis, and tendon balancing is a necessary part of the correction. This concept is logical. The cause of every cavus foot is the result of muscle imbalance; therefore, why should an arthrodesis, even a triple arthrodesis, be sufficient to correct and then maintain correction of the deformity if muscle imbalance is still present? The PTT inserts distal to the talonavicular joint, and unless the PTT is transferred, the medial foot deformity gradually recurs, with onset of adductovarus. Therefore, if a

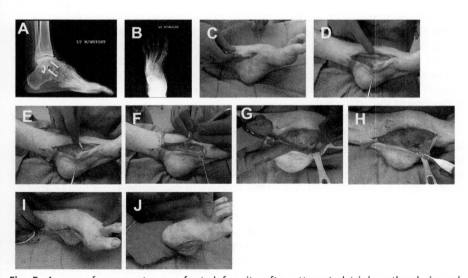

Fig. 5. A case of recurrent cavus foot deformity after attempted triple arthrodesis and without any soft tissue balancing procedure. Note the persistent cavus and varus deformity of the midfoot (*A, B*). In the revision surgery, a PTT transfer (*C, D*) and an abductor fascia (*E, F*) and plantar fascia release (*G, H*) were performed. Note the midfoot adduction deformity was remarkably corrected after the soft tissue balancing procedures (*I, J*).

triple arthrodesis is believed the procedure of choice, it should be performed with appropriate transfer of the PTT. There are cavus feet where there is no adductovarus deformity present, and there is a global severe midfoot cavus with rotation of the midfoot (equinus) of the first metatarsal and rotation of the lateral column. In these cases where the predominant deforming force is the strong peroneus longus and a weak anterior tibial muscle, the PTT still can be used to augment the power of dorsiflexion with a transfer through the interosseous membrane to the dorsum of the foot. In the same example, the peroneus longus should be transferred into the peroneus brevis to decrease the force on the medial forefoot.

For correction of severe hindfoot deformities, the traditional procedure for decades has been a triple arthrodesis or various modifications of this procedure; however, the literature from the 1970s indicated that a triple arthrodesis was not associated with long-term success in the cavus foot. Santavirta and colleagues[11] reviewed 15 consecutive patients treated for Charcot-Marie-Tooth (CMT) disease, of whom 21 were treated with triple arthrodesis. Six of these feet underwent simultaneous soft tissue procedures, and 5 feet in 3 patients needed subsequent additional soft tissue procedures to improve foot balance after healing.[11] Wukich and Bowen[12] followed 34 feet that underwent triple arthrodesis for pes cavus and reported that 22 of the feet had continued pain and 19 feet had plantar callosities. They noted that residual deformity, including cavus, varus, and cavovarus, was present in 15 of 34 feet (45%). They commented and support the authors' hypothesis that a fusion cannot be relied on without balancing the muscular forces. Even with a well-performed triple arthrodesis, there are still forces on the midfoot, such as the tibialis posterior, tibialis anterior, and peroneus longus imbalance, and the long extensors, which if left in place, continue to act as deforming forces. Wetmore and Drennan[13] reported on 30 feet in 16 patients for an average of 21 years and reported 30% fair and 47% poor results, with persistent varus and cavus noted in 9 feet and recurrence of cavovarus occurred in 7 feet (23%) that had originally been correctly aligned. They recommended that a triple arthrodesis should be performed with muscle-balancing procedures to reduce the risk of recurrence. The results of this study should serve as a warning to the surgeon who plans to rely on bony correction alone for the cavus foot, and each of these studies, discussed previously, demonstrates what is bound to happen without the addition of soft tissue balancing, that is, tendon transfer. The authors strongly believe that these types of outcomes can be avoided when the appropriate tendon transfer is performed at the time of the arthrodesis.

When approaching the rigid cavus deformity, it is possible to perform an anatomic correction of the foot initially, even with a triple arthrodesis, but this procedure is insufficient in the long term if muscular imbalance remains. Integral to the success of any of these procedures is a corrected foot posture, a plantigrade hindfoot relative to the forefoot, and muscle balance. Even with perfectly executed surgery, if the posterior tibial muscle is overactive relative to the evertors of the hindfoot, the foot ultimately will fail, with further adductovarus deformity. The posterior tibial muscle, therefore, must be transferred in many if not most of these procedures. Frequently, a cavus deformity is associated with slight weakness of the anterior tibial muscle, and the PTT can be transferred as part of this corrective procedure. Usually, the transfer, therefore, is made through the interosseous membrane to the dorsum of the foot. If the anterior tibial muscle is strong and the predominant deformity is adductovarus, then the peroneus longus is transferred into the peroneus brevis tendon, but the deforming force of the posterior tibial muscle must still be considered, and at times this too is transferred and inserted more laterally, that is, in the cuboid, to maintain correction of deformity.[5,14,15]

The peroneus longus-to-brevis tendon transfer is a useful procedure when the peroneus longus muscle is working and is flexible, which is the usual situation, whether a flexible or a rigid cavus foot. Regardless of the strength of the peroneus brevis tendon, this transfer augments the weak peroneus brevis muscle. Ideally, this procedure is done in younger patients and even in children to achieve maximal advantage or when the foot is more flexible. Surgeon must be careful using this transfer in young patients to augment the eversion strength when a PTT transfer is performed simultaneously in the absence of a hindfoot arthrodesis.

It is always essential to keep in mind the principles of correction of a cavus foot deformity, because, as discussed previously, muscle balance must be obtained. In some patients, this requirement is obvious, because they have a paralytic deformity, such as a foot drop, in addition to the cavus deformity. The authors try to use whatever tendon is available, in particular whichever muscle is a deforming force on the foot and ankle. This applies to the extensor hallucis longus, the extensor digitorum longus, the PTT, the peroneus longus, and any other tendon that may be used to correct deformity.

A MULTIPLANAR DEFORMITY IS PRESENT

It is not common to have a foot that is simply deformed in the sagittal plane, that is, a cavus is present, regardless of the apex of the deformity. In addition to the cavus, the hindfoot is always in varus and the midfoot supinated and also adducted. In addition to these deformities, there may be varying degrees of equinus as a result of a contracture of either the Achilles or the gastrocnemius soleus complex, hence the terms, cavus, cavovarus, cavo-adductovarus, and cavo-equinovarus. Whatever is done to correct 1 plane of deformity has an impact on the other planes. The obvious example of this is that when moving a varus hindfoot deformity into valgus, the medial column moves into more plantarflexion. This concept applies to all cavus deformity corrections, particular in multiplanar deformity, that is, where there are multiple apices of the deformity.[5,16,17]

A triple arthrodesis and its variants have been the mainstay of correction of the hindfoot deformity, but it has to be appreciated that a triple arthrodesis as an isolated procedure is never sufficient for correction of severe multiplanar deformity. As discussed previously, a tendon transfer must always be performed and then additional procedures, including midfoot or forefoot osteotomy or arthrodesis, to balance the foot and create a plantigrade surface for weight bearing. Wetmore and Drennan[13] reported that a high failure of triple arthrodesis in many patients was the development of recurrent deformity as well as development of ankle arthritis. The authors believe, however, that a triple arthrodesis is a good procedure, provided that the foot is correctly balanced with additional osteotomy and tendon transfers as needed. The triple arthrodesis gained a poor reputation for correction of the cavus foot, in particular that associated with CMT. These arthrodesis procedures were performed in isolation, and, as might be expected, the deformity recurred. Correction of multiplanar deformity probably is one of the more difficult orthopedic foot and ankle procedures to perform. Not only is the structural deformity associated with bone deformity in multiple planes but also joint contractures and muscle imbalance are other factors that must be addressed. As discussed previously, the approach to correction of this type of deformity involves structural bone alteration in conjunction with adequate muscle and soft tissue balancing (**Fig. 6**).

AN ADDUCTOVARUS DEFORMITY IS PRESENT

This is a more severe variant of the cavus foot, which can be an adductus of the midfoot associated with varus of the hindfoot or adductus associated with hindfoot varus

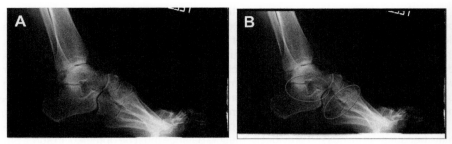

Fig. 6. A case of severe cavus foot deformity (*A*). Note the multiple plane deformities in both the subtalar joint and the TMT joint (*B*). Also, the approach to correction of this type of deformity involves both structural bone alteration, in conjunction with adequate muscle and soft tissue balancing.

and forefoot cavus as well as equinus (**Fig. 7**). This is a variant of severe deformity and, much as described previously, this includes correction of the more severe multiplanar deformity.[18] The only difference is that in addition to the transfer of the PTT, there may be severe contracture of the medial soft tissues, including the abductor hallucis fascia, which also requires release. Once the PTT has been detached and the plantar fascia and abductor fascia cut, then the arthrodesis procedures continue but with a slightly different approach to include a resection of a lateral wedge from the calcaneocuboid joint.

THE MIDFOOT IS SUPINATED AND THE FIFTH METATARSAL FIXED AND ROTATED UNDER THE CUBOID

Beware of the patient with a significant callosity under the base of the fifth metatarsal. This is always associated with a severe hindfoot varus and supination of the midfoot and also at times associated with adduction of the midfoot. A sizable callus is present and sometimes there may even have been prior episodes of ulceration over the base of the fifth metatarsal. On radiographs the metatarsals appear so rotated that the base

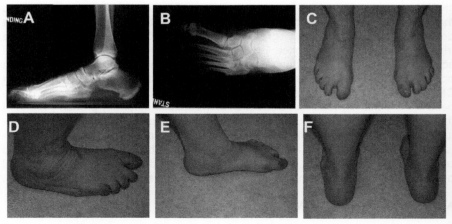

Fig. 7. A case of adductovarus foot (*B, C, D, E*). Note the alignment of the hindfoot is acceptable (*F*), whereas the midfoot is in adductus (*B*) and varus deformity (*A*).

of the fifth metatarsal is not visible on the anteroposterior view. The fifth metatarsal is markedly depressed relative to the first metatarsal, and in more severe deformities it lies inferior to the plane of the cuboid. Other radiographic markers of cavus deformity are evident, but in the patients with lateral column overload, the fifth metatarsal always assumes a position in which it is rotated and closer to the ground than the other rays.

For these deformities, after the triple arthrodesis, with wedge resection of the lateral subtalar joint to correct the hindfoot varus combined with a lateral wedge through the calcaneocuboid joint, the lateral side of the foot generally corrects. After complete joint preparation, the hindfoot is moved into valgus, and the adduction and supination of the transverse tarsal joint are accomplished by removing a wedge from the calcaneocuboid joint and then pushing up on the cuboid to ensure that there is no residual pressure under the fifth metatarsal. This assumes, however, that the fifth metatarsal will move with the cuboid, but, for severe rigid deformities, the fifth metatarsal is fixed under the cuboid and this does not take place.

With these types of deformity, ostectomy or resection of the base of the fifth metatarsal is necessary, although many patients still have sensation, and the deformity of fifth metatarsal can be more than just a nuisance with callosity but also painful. Nonetheless, to achieve better correction with a more plantigrade foot, ostectomy of the fifth metatarsal is a good procedure and can be done in conjunction with any additional necessary procedure. The lateral incision of the triple arthrodesis is extended distally along the lateral border of the fifth metatarsal shaft while staying slightly dorsal to the plantar skin. Once the base of the fifth metatarsal is adequately exposed, the ostectomy is performed with a saw. The orientation of the ostectomy is biplanar with the blade angled from dorsal-lateral to plantar-medial in the coronal plane and from proximal-dorsal to distal-plantar in the sagittal plane to create a beveled cut. The metatarsal base is then grasped with a towel clamp and its soft tissue attachments, including the peroneus brevis and short plantar ligament, are sharply dissected away for completion of the ostectomy. It is important that at the completion of the osteotomy, no bone prominence remains on the plantar lateral weight-bearing surface. For this reason, it may even be necessary to shave the under surface of the cuboid after resection of the base of the fifth metatarsal.[19]

The peroneus brevis tendon can be detached distally because it is generally nonfunctional with these more severe deformities, in particular those associated with CMT. This depends, however, on the stability of the ankle. If the peroneus brevis needs to be used as part of an ankle ligament reconstruction, this can still be done by suturing the attachment of the tendon distally to the periosteum and the surrounding tissue, even supplementing the attachment with a suture anchor into the cuboid. If the peroneus brevis is irreparably torn or absent, then the peroneus longus or a free tendon graft can be used for the ankle ligament reconstruction.

REFERENCES

1. Aminian A, Sangeorzan BJ. The anatomy of caves foot deformity. Foot Ankle Clin 2008;13:191–8.
2. Paley D. Principles of deformity correction. Berlin: Springer-Verlag; 2002.
3. Perera A, Guha A. Clinical and radiographic evaluation of the cavus foot: surgical implications. Foot Ankle Clin 2013;18(4):619–28.
4. Zide JR, Myerson MS. Arthrodesis for the cavus foot: when, where, and how? Foot Ankle Clin 2013;18(4):755–67.
5. Sammarco GJ, Taylor R. Combined calcaneal and metatarsal osteotomies for the treatment of caves foot. Foot Ankle Clin 2001;6:533–43.

6. Jahss MH. Tarsometatarsal truncated-wedge arthrodesis for pes cavus and equinovarus deformity of the fore part of the foot. J Bone Joint Surg Am. 1980;62(5): 713–22.

7. Wulker N, Hurschler C. Cavus foot correction in adults by dorsal closing wedge osteotomy. Foot Ankle Int 2002;23:344–7.

8. Huber M. What is role of tendon transfer in the caves foot? Foot Ankle Clin 2013;4: 689–95.

9. Krause FG, Wing KJ, Younger AS. Neuromuscular issues in cavovarus foot. Foot Ankle Clin 2008;13:243–58.

10. Ward CM, Dolan LA, Bennett DL, et al. Long-term results of reconstruction for treatment of a flexible cavovarus foot in Charcot-Marie-Tooth disease. J Bone Joint Surg Am 2008;90:2631–42.

11. Santavirta S, Turunen V, Ylinen P, et al. Foot and ankle fusions in Charcot-Marie-Tooth disease. Arch Orthop Trauma Surg 1993;112(4):175–9.

12. Wukich DK, Bowen JR. A long-term study of triple arthrodesis for correction of pes cavovarus in Charcot-Marie-Tooth disease. J Pediatr Orthop 1989;9(4): 433–7.

13. Wetmore RS, Drennan JC. Long-term results of triple arthrodesis in Charcot-Marie-Tooth disease. J Bone Joint Surg Am 1989;71(3):417–22.

14. Dreher T, Wolf SI, Heitzmann D, et al. Tibialis posterior tendon transfer corrects the foot drop component of cavovarus foot deformity in Charcot-Marie-Tooth disease. J Bone Joint Surg Am 2014;96(6):456–62.

15. Steinau HU, Tofaute A, Huellmann K, et al. Tendon transfers for drop foot correction: long-term results including quality of life assessment, and dynamometric and pedobarographic measurements. Arch Orthop Trauma Surg 2011;131(7): 903–10.

16. Joseph TN, Myerson MS. Correction of multiplanar hindfoot deformity with osteotomy, arthrodesis, and internal fixation. Instr Course Lect 2005;54:269–76.

17. Bishay SN. Single-event multilevel acute total correction of complex equinocavovarus deformity in skeletally mature patients with spastic cerebral palsy hemiparesis. J Foot Ankle Surg 2013;52(4):481–5.

18. Pentz AS, Weiner DS. Management of metatarsus adductovarus. Foot Ankle 1993;14(5):241–6.

19. Shariff R, Myerson MS, Palmanovich E. Resection of the fifth metatarsal base in the severe rigid cavovarus foot. Foot Ankle Int 2014;35(6):558–65.

Moving?

Make sure your subscription moves with you!

To notify us of your new address, find your **Clinics Account Number** (located on your mailing label above your name), and contact customer service at:

Email: journalscustomerservice-usa@elsevier.com

800-654-2452 (subscribers in the U.S. & Canada)
314-447-8871 (subscribers outside of the U.S. & Canada)

Fax number: 314-447-8029

Elsevier Health Sciences Division
Subscription Customer Service
3251 Riverport Lane
Maryland Heights, MO 63043

*To ensure uninterrupted delivery of your subscription, please notify us at least 4 weeks in advance of move.

Printed and bound by CPI Group (UK) Ltd, Croydon, CR0 4YY

08/05/2025

01864745-0003